Exceed The Feed Limit!

Out of The Fat Lane Into A Slimmer, Healthier Life Without Diets Or Deprivation

Vicki Park

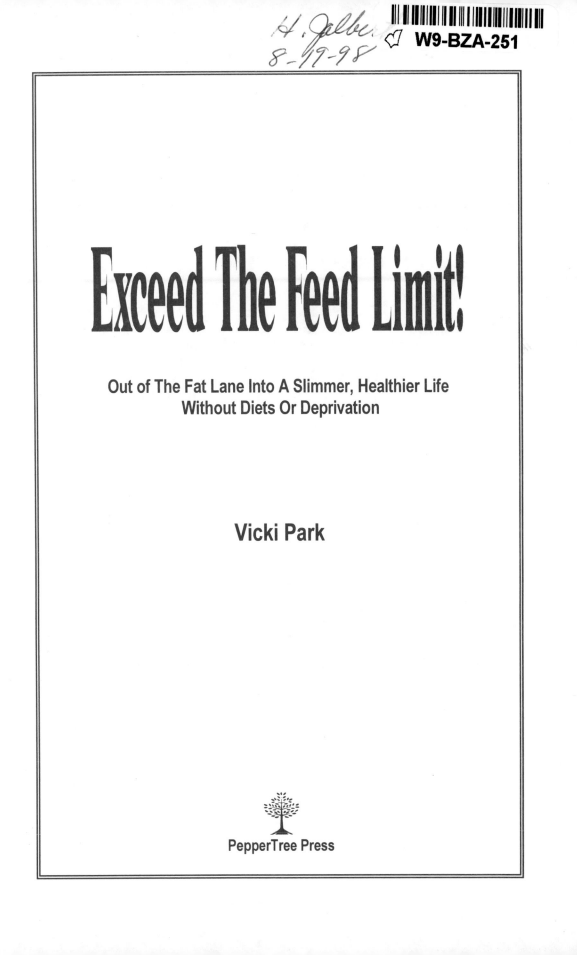

PepperTree Press

Published by: PepperTree Press
Post Office Box 232
Pleasant Grove, Alabama 35127

ISBN 0-9642733-1-4
Library of Congress Catalog Card Number 96-71399

Cover Photography: Spider Martin
Cover Design: Roger M. Mortensen

An Important Reminder

This book is based upon the author's own personal experience and opinions. It is not intended to replace the advice of a medical professional. Before starting any eating program, weight loss program or exercise program, it is vital to receive the permission and recommendation of your physician.

Dedication

This book is especially dedicated to Jo Ellen O'Hara, whose wonderful writing I have always admired and who made my career as a writer a Cinderella story; to Gary Wright, who gave me the publicity that most writers only get to dream about and to everyone at Warner Books, Oxmoor House and Pepper-Tree Press. It is also dedicated to my terrific family and to the memory of my father, Virgil Whatley, my mother-in-law, Odell Park and our friend Van Davis, as well as to all those wonderful friends and readers who have been so supportive and marvelous. I love you all.

Special Thanks

There is no way that words can express my appreciation for the assistance that so many people have given me. In truth, this list of those I would like to thank should be longer than this entire book. However, in the interest of brevity, I will just say thank you from the bottom of my heart to all of you who have helped me with my books, videos and other projects. In addition, I would like to especially thank my husband, Ken; my daughter, Ashley; my Mom, Lorene Whatley; Elmer Park; Lou and Buddy Renfroe; Jan Moore; Mike Dulin; Irma and Joe Thomas; Kelli Agnew; Joe M. Thomas; Gina and Roy Bradley; Gary Wright; Carolyn Smith; Lane Schmidt; Ruthann Essinger; Gary Brown; Mark Mortensen; Spider Martin; Christina Todd; Amy Gary; Helen Davis; Linda Mendel; Brenda Gill; Helen and Charles Horton; Lorraine Walker; Virginia Guthrie; Richard Manoske; Sam Granger; Doris Odom; Ann Isaac and her wonderful team; Dr. Jimmy Bridges; Bruce Martin; Wanda Barton; Edith Harwell and the Homewood Library staff; Ann Scott; Norma Owen; Scott Moreland; Pat Pisanos; Randy West; Brenda Self; Kathryn Kaufman; Martha Chandler; Sue Harrison; Gwen Maness; Archie and Sharon Phillips; Keith Dempsey; William Capps; Joan Colvert; Wanda Wheeler; Gerry Wheeler; Judy Clark; Margaret Glasscock; Joe Guin; Ted Hipp; David John; Kate Cozart; Milt Kahn and Sandra Brown. Thank you all more than words can say.

Contents
A Little Inspiration And A Lot Of Information

Contents

Section Three: The Recipes (Continued)

Preface

Y ou never know where or when you may learn something profound about yourself. It can sometimes happen in the most unexpected places. Some years ago I found myself driving down a narrow, winding road behind a huge motor home. It was barely moving. I was on my way to work and I just knew it was going to make me late.

The owner of the motor home was rather thoughtful. To entertain those forced to creep along behind him, he had covered the whole back end with bumper stickers, which were mainly of the "I owe, I owe, it's off to work I go" school of terrible puns. Normally, I'm a sucker for puns. The cornier the better. My husband often threatens to call the imaginary pun police to come get me because I'm always telling some real groaners.

However, that day I was so anxious about getting to work on time that the bumper stickers didn't do much to cheer me. Then I spotted one that didn't just make me smile, it changed my life. It was from that little bumper sticker that I learned the reason I had never been able to stick to a diet.

I always figured the inability to lose weight was some sort of character flaw on my part. I probably hold the record for the world's shortest diets. I would frequently get out of bed promising myself to start a new diet and change my mind by the time I opened my refrigerator door two minutes later. Even if I managed to hang in there for a while, in the long run I always ended up weighing more than when I started.

At the time I saw the bumper sticker, I had "dieted" my way up to 315 pounds. I considered myself a hopeless failure at weight loss. But that little bumper sticker finally explained to me in a few short words why diets had never worked for me. It simply said: A DIET IS THE PUNISHMENT FOR EXCEEDING THE FEED LIMIT! Okay, stop groaning. Maybe you want to call the pun police about that one, but just think about it for a minute. Truer words were never written.

It isn't just me who can relate to that bit of roadside psychology. It applies to all of us who have never been able to stick to a diet. From what some of the experts tell us, that is just about everybody who ever tried. They also tell us that even if we do manage to lose we probably won't be able to permanently keep it off. We are programmed by news like that to expect failure.

But wait! We have that good old bumper sticker to explain to us why that happens. A DIET IS THE PUNISHMENT FOR EXCEEDING THE FEED LIMIT! There it is in a nutshell. When we diet, we are punishing ourselves. By limiting ourselves to tiny portions of tasteless foods, by subjecting ourselves to weighing and measuring each morsel and by condemning ourselves to constant hunger, we are punishing ourselves for overeating—for exceeding the feed limit. Since no one in their right mind enjoys punishment, few people are willing to keep punishing themselves for long. We are usually back to eating as usual within a very short time. Who can blame us since eating is one of the great pleasures of life?

I have joked about the pun police but they are nothing compared to those imaginary diet police who place us under arrest for overeating and sentence us to rabbit food for life. I named this book *Exceed The Feed Limit!* because the words in the title are true. We don't have to fear failure or punishment by the diet police any more just because we enjoy eating.

Things are changing. There have been exciting developments in the fields of weight loss and nutrition. Researchers now realize that it is possible to lose weight without deprivation or dieting. It can be simply a matter of controlling the amount of fat we eat and the type of food we eat.

When you lower the amount of fat that you eat, you often can, with certain exceptions, eat more food than you could eat on an old-fashioned calorie-based diet and still lose weight. I am living proof. When I stopped dieting I lost 180 pounds. Not only that, my husband Ken lost 90 pounds. We've kept the weight off for six years. Our daughter Ashley has lost the 85 pounds she gained at college too. We never had to give up hearty portions of our favorite dishes—we just learned to enjoy them in a healthier way.

I am not a doctor or nutritionist but I do have something to share that I think can be helpful too—personal experience. By distilling the wisdom I learned from medical experts into a simple system that fit into my busy lifestyle, I finally found a way to lose weight without dieting or deprivation. I had to pass along the good news in hopes that it could help others. As a result I wrote a book called *Live! Don't Diet!*

Live! Don't Diet! has sold more than 120,000 copies and has led to my appearance on TV and radio shows, as well as to stories in newspapers and magazines across the country. The reaction to *Live! Don't Diet!* surpassed my wildest dreams. However, the most exciting thing is not the attention it has received from the media, it is the wonderful letters I have received from people who have told me the book has helped them lose weight and eat healthier too. That gives me joy beyond measure.

Whether or not you have read *Live! Don't Diet!* I hope you'll find *Exceed The Feed Limit!* a helpful addition to your kitchen. You may want to lose weight or perhaps you just want eat healthier. In either case, I have written it especially for you.

It contains 200 quick and easy low-fat recipes that have helped me, Ken and Ashley lose 355 pounds and keep it off. I hope you'll like my recipes. They are quick, simple and made with ingredients that you don't have to go across town to buy. In fact you probably already have many of the ingredients in your pantry. The recipes are not delicacies that require a gourmet or chef to prepare. They are simple, hearty dishes because that is what we like to eat at our houseand these are the recipes I prepare every day.

In addition to my recipes, *Exceed The Feed Limit!* also contains lots of information about eating low-fat, as well as some words that I hope will inspire and motivate you. I hope you will enjoy and benefit from the recipes, tips and techniques I have included. A better life is just a meal away. So come along with me—the best is yet to be!

Section One
A Little Inspiration

Let's Get Motivated!

I am not only here to share my recipes and weight loss tips, I am also here to inspire and motivate you. After all, motivation is a major part of successful weight loss. It is very simple—if you aren't motivated, you probably won't succeed. Remember that it's the brain that tells you to open your mouth and shovel that rich, fattening dessert in! It is also the brain that tells you how wonderful you will look and feel when you don't give in to temptation. The trick is to train your brain to think the latter way instead of the former. That's motivation!

It is so important to have some compelling reason you want to lose or improve your eating habits. Maybe it's to live a longer life and to look better and feel better. Heaven knows, there couldn't be any more important reasons. But sometimes it takes more personal reasons. I wanted to be able to have more fun in life and to wear shorts or a bathing suit without embarassment. Call them vain reasons but they worked for me. The mind is the master of the body. That's the reason coaches give pep talks to their teams before a big game. Motivation works. It keeps you focused. So get your mind in gear and go out and win this one for you!

On the next few pages I want to share a few more words to inspire you. Whenever you need a boost to your motivation, go back and re-read them. Also look at the before and after pictures of me on the cover. I am living proof it can be done. The weight I lost made such a dramatic difference in my life yet I didn't have to do anything but make some easy changes in the way I cook and eat. Such a simple thing changed and probably saved my life.

Because I began cooking healthier, Ken also lost the weight he needed to lose and was able to stop taking cholesterol and blood pressure medication. So, you see, it's not just ourselves, it's other members of our family we may be helping. Helping family members improve their health and weight can be a powerful inspiration in itself. So, come on. We'll get and keep your mind on track! Your body has only to follow!

Don't Just Dream It...Do It!

I am a real creature of habit. I really don't like changes in my lifestyle very much. When my daily routine varies very much from the norm, it throws me into a tailspin. I may never retire from the job I have held for almost 30 years because I'm afraid that I could never adjust to a more leisurely routine after years of going to work every day. I'm also afraid I would start putting everything off.

I am a world class procrastinator. I'm like the guy who bought a book titled *Stop Putting Things Off!* but never got around to reading it. If I ever did retire I could probably keep busy finishing up all those half completed craft projects now littering my basement but I would probably end up putting that off too.

I am glad to know I'm not alone in my penchant for procrastination. A friend whose husband shares this same trait used to swear that there was nothing he wouldn't put off. One day she came in with an amazed expression on her face. "Well," she said. "I guess I'll have to eat my words. I have been after Jim for months to fix that shaky old TV antenna on our roof but he never would. Yesterday, during the windstorm, it blew down right in the middle of the football game he was watching. He leapt up, ran to the closet, grabbed a wire coathanger, dragged the TV out onto the front porch, stuck the coathanger into the back of the TV and watched the rest of the game!"

I guess the point here is that sometimes we have to be galvanized into action whether we want to be or not. We may have been told by a doctor that we have to lose weight or that we must change our eating habits for health reasons. We may do it because we need to feel better. Sadly, we may feel we have to do it to keep the affections of someone we love. There can be loads of reasons. In my case, I just didn't want to let fat rob me of the fun and excitement of life anymore. However, as I mentioned I don't like change. I am also a selfish person. While I wanted to be thinner, I obviously didn't want to have to go to much trouble to do it. I didn't like being fat but I also didn't want to punish my-self.

People are always saying to me, "You must have had terri-fic willpower to have lost all that weight." Honestly I never had any willpower and I still don't. If this way had not been the easi-est I had ever tried, I still would weigh 315 pounds—or more. I simply learned to cook the things I love to eat in a healthier way. I still cook the same things I always cooked, I still eat a lot of food and I still don't have to spend much time in the kitchen.

More about all that later. I'll give you the details in the section called "The Basics Of Low-Fat Weight Loss". Mean-while, there is another point I want to make. We all have goals and dreams that we never get around to pursuing. We either de-cide they are too much trouble or we let other things in life get in our way. Don't let it happen to you. Whether it is weight loss or another goal you have put off pursuing—get started on it now. You never know where it may lead. When I made the decision to try to lose weight again and sat down at my kitchen table to re-duce the fat in my recipes, I never dreamed that I would lose 180 pounds or become a cookbook author.

When I was a child we were required to memorize poetry in school. That is so long ago that I barely remember the name of the school I attended, but I do remember part of one of the po-ems. It was called Maude Muller by John Greenleaf Whittier and the lines were these:

"Of all the sad words of tongue or pen
The saddest are these: It might have been."

I didn't want to come to the end of my days and wonder what life might have been like if I had only gotten my weight un-der control. Don't let that happen to you either. Whether it's do-ing something about your weight or some other goal you have put off pursuing—**DON'T JUST DREAM ABOUT IT! DO IT!** You'll be glad you did.

Taking Stock:
A Blueprint For Your Future

What if you lived in an house that you had not cared for as well as you should have. As a result, things are starting to go wrong. The exterior is getting a little shabby and the plumbing is starting to go bad. What if you had the opportunity to remodel your home into a better, more attractive one—at no cost and with very little effort? Anyone who wouldn't jump at the chance to do that would be considered crazy! You have the same opportunity with your body. After all your body is the earthly home your soul inhabits and you should want to make that home a mansion.

There are very few people who couldn't use a little self improvement. We all could do with a little remodeling once in a while. Take stock of yourself. Would you like to be the person you always dreamed you could be? Would you like to live life in a body that is healthier and more attractive? Why settle for just "being" when with so little effort you could be the best that you can be.

It isn't vain to want to look and feel your best. It is only sensible. Just as blueprints are used to remodel a house, you can draw up the blueprints for a new you. Take stock of yourself. What would you like to change? Consider the following questions:

- Are you overweight? Even five pounds can make a difference in the way you look and feel and may affect your life span.

- Are you suffering from the effects of an unhealthy diet? Do you have high blood pressure or cholesterol problems or feel that you are at risk for developing illnesses that may be diet-related?

- Have you let your attitude about life slowly grow more and more negative? Are you seldom enthusiastic about the events going on in your life?

- Have you grown stagnant in your relationships with others— and with yourself?

- Does your appearance need upgrading? Is your wardrobe more of a cover-up than an enhancement?

If the answer to any of the above questions is even "maybe" you could probably benefit from a little personal re-modeling. A really good place to start is with your eating habits. It is amazing how the foods we allow ourselves to eat can affect so many facets of our lives. Just think about it. The guilt we face when we overeat or eat things that are bad for us, the weight we may gain, the health problems we may engender, can affect everything we do. Food is a major thread in the physical and emotional fabric of our lives.

By beginning to eat healthier, you may be taking the first baby steps toward a whole new you. As you eat better, you begin to feel better. As you feel better, you want to look better. As you look better, your self-esteem and your enthusiasm for life increases. As your self esteem and enthusiasm increases, your relationships with the people in your life may improve. One step leads to another. I speak from experience. That is exactly what happened to me.

Change taken in small steps is so gradual that it seems almost effortless. It can be a tremendous gift to those you love when you become the best that you can be—but it is really a gift you are giving yourself. When you are looking and feeling your best, you are usually happier and less stressed. You are not only emotionally healthier, you are generally physically healthier as well. Self improvement is literally a gift to yourself that can last a lifetime—a happier and quite possibly a longer lifetime. So get started now remodeling yourself and before long you will be the "you" of your dreams.

Is There Time And Energy For Fun In Your Life?

I have never seen a tombstone yet that said: "She Kept Her House Perfectly Cleaned" or "She Spent All Of Her Time In The Kitchen." I bet you haven't either. Somehow those things lose their importance in the grand scheme of things.

Of course it is important to keep our homes clean and our families well fed, but often we have a tendency to equate the amount of time we spend on these things with being a worthwhile person. This could be due in large part to the barrage of commercials that imply that a truly worthwhile person has a floor that shines like a mirror and demonstrates love by providing a constant supply of fat-laden homemade goodies. Many of us have become slaves to this concept. As a result, we are too overworked and worn out to enjoy life.

I must admit, I bought into the concept, too. While I never was one to spend much time in the kitchen, I did find myself feeling very guilty if I didn't try to keep my house in perfect condition. I hate even the most routine housework, yet I made myself spend endless hours doing extra household tasks that were noticeable to no one but me. Trying to work full time, raise a teenager and keep a perfect home left me very tired and usually grumpy. Considering that I also weighed 315 pounds, I am amazed that I ever smiled.

One day, it occurred to me that I had let being a super cleaner become so important to me because it gave me back some of the self-esteem that I had allowed fat to take from me. It allowed me to control some aspect of my life. I weighed 315 pounds, so obviously I couldn't control my appetite, but I could control my house. I may have gotten some self-esteem from this, but it didn't make me happy because I really hated doing those household tasks.

Once I started my low-fat lifestyle, began losing weight and gained control over that very important aspect of my life, being a cleaning dynamo didn't seem quite so important anymore. It no longer bothers me if my floors don't sparkle, as long as they are clean. Now, I spend the time I used to spend on extra housekeeping tasks with my husband or my daughter. It is amazing the difference it has made in the atmosphere in our home. We are all happier because Mom isn't so grumpy anymore.

The point of my dime store psychoanalysis is this: if you too have been brainwashed into believing that you must have the perfectly cleaned home or must demonstrate your love by endless hours of baking rich treats for your family, just think about it for a minute. No one is really comfortable in a perfect home—and feeding your family great dishes that are good for them spells loving more than any fat-laden, sugary junk.

Unless you really love extra cleaning or spending all of your time in the kitchen, don't feel guilty about not doing it. Spend that time in doing things with those you love. Memories are not made from perfectly kept homes, they are made from having fun with people we care about. If you do really love cleaning, at least make the arrangements to get "She Kept Her House Perfectly Cleaned" carved on your tombstone. That's the only thing about housework that will last!

I've Been Fat And I've Been Thin

To paraphrase that old line "I've been rich and I've been poor and rich is better," I'd like to say that I've been fat and I've been thinner—and thinner is better. I guess the politically correct term might be weight challenged while the feel good term of the moment for obesity is fluffy, but I wasn't weight challenged or fluffy—I was downright fat!

I know that there are many happy, heavy people who may beg to differ, but having seen the issue from both sides, I have many reasons to personally feel that being thinner is infinitely better. Here's just a few of the reasons:

- I used to catch every cold that came within a city block of me when I was heavy. It probably had more to do with my eating habits than my size, but now that I have lost weight, eat healthy and am more active, I haven't had a cold in years.

- Speaking of being active, when I was heavy, I just didn't have the energy to be very active. Now that I have lost weight, I have more energy than I had as a teenager. It is a great feeling.

- When my husband and I were heavy, a substantial portion of our income went toward buying blood pressure and cholesterol-lowering medications. Because we lost weight and eat healthier, we no longer have to take any of those medications. Now we have better health plus more spending money!

- I used to suffer with chronic knee and ankle pain from carrying around excess weight. Several heavy friends of mine actually had to have knee surgery because of problems associated with overweight. After I lost weight, all of my joint pain ended.

- When I was heavy, I couldn't cross my legs because they were too large. They say that some of life's greatest pleasures are the simplest. For me, finally being able to sit with my legs crossed was such a terrific moment. It may sound silly, but unless you have had the same problem yourself, you can't imagine how uncomfortable it can be to never be able to cross your legs.

- When I was heavy, I stayed drenched with perspiration from May until October. Just thinking of that sticky, awful feeling makes me shudder.

- Once, when I was heavy, it took two brave, strong men to hoist me into a horse-drawn carriage in New Orleans. When I finally got in, I couldn't fit into the seat. A friend once told me she was mega-embarassed when she had to leave a boat because the life vest was too small to fit her.

- I used to envy the cool, comfortable women I would see dressed in shorts during the summer. I wore heavy gabardine slacks, mainly because they covered up a lot. What's more, they were usually black because I thought I looked smaller in black. Talk about hot! Granted, I should have dressed in shorts and not have cared a fig about the opinions of anyone else, but I am ashamed to say that I was superficial when it came to the opinions of others.

- Once, when I attended a meeting, the chairperson announced "Before we get started, I am sure Vicki would like to know where the snack machines are located in the building." I have been lucky. Many heavy people have been the victims of considerably worse remarks.

I could go on and on with examples, but I think you get the idea. These are just some very minor examples of the personal ways being overweight impacted my life. In retrospect, I was very fortunate to not have experienced severe problems. Obviously there could have been some, such as very serious or even life-threatening illness. So many very severe health problems are linked to overweight and to fat in the diet.

If you don't have control of your eating, some of these problems may become your problems if they are not already. I can assure you that the momentary pleasure of unlimited amounts of fattening food is not worth the many problems that being overweight can cause.

Here's To Your Good Health!

If you have had any exposure to a newspaper or a news program today, I would be willing to bet that you saw a story on the damage that eating too much fat can do to the body. Few days go by without new, alarming revelations about it. Dietary fat has been implicated as the culprit in an enormous number of health problems. We all know about heart disease and a wide variety of cancers, but now scientists are even linking it to such unexpected diseases as certain types of blindness. Apparently there is no part of the body that cannot be damaged by eating too much fat. In fact, it has been noted that most premature deaths caused by illness can be linked to diet—and especially dietary fat.

Of course one of the biggest problems (another bad pun—please excuse me!) too much dietary fat can cause is obesity. If a day passes without a news story on another disease that excessive fat intake can cause, there is sure to be a story on the perils of being overweight. Recent studies have indicated that even being slightly overweight can cut years from your life span. What a terrible thought. Not only are we doomed if we eat too much fat, we also are doomed if we are overweight at all.

Even if you or members of your family are as thin as a rail, the amount of fat that you eat can do great harm to you. The skinniest person I know has terrible cholesterol and blood pressure problems, mainly because she mainlines cheeseburgers and fatty junk foods. I'm sure you know someone just like her. Everyone does. They're the people we love to hate but secretly envy because they seem to be able to eat enormous quantities of the most fattening foods without gaining an ounce. One of their favorite expressions is, "Well, I don't have to worry about what I eat. I can eat anything I want to." This statement is usually delivered with an air of gleeful superiority. I have heard it a million times. Well, it may seem that they are immune but it will probably catch up with them some day. Even people who are a perfect size need to eat healthier or they may be taking years off their life.

Of course, what you drink can be just as important as what you eat. You no doubt recognize the title of this segment as a classic toast, but when toasting your good health, do it with a non-alcoholic drink. Drinking alcohol, especially before or during meals, can lower willpower and make you more susceptible to eating what you want instead of what you know you should have. In other words, that high-fat prime rib or favorite ultra-rich dish in the restaurant may not be so easy to turn down after a little alcohol is in your system. It make's sense. If alcohol lowers other inhibitions, why not those involving food?

Researchers are now saying that it is never too late to improve our health by improving our eating habits. Don't just sit there contemplating whether your spouse will bring a date to your funeral. As the old saying goes—stop digging your grave with your knife and fork! It has never been easier to eat low-fat. The food industry has seen the handwriting on the wall and seldom a day goes by without a great new low-fat product in the grocery store. You can eat healthy and also lose weight with an ease you never dreamed possible.

Lower The Fat And Raise The Roof!

Once, when I weighed 315 pounds, I sat in the car for 6 hours rather than join my family as they hiked a beautiful trail in the Smoky mountains. While they enjoyed quality time together, I dozed, alone and miserable. That is what fat will do for you. I am not just talking about fat on the body, I am also talking about fat in the body. Even people who are of average weight can feel sluggish and dull when they consume too much fat. It can make even the simple movments of our everyday routine seem tiring.

I have received numerous letters from people of all sizes who tell me how much better they feel now that they have reduced the amount of fat they are consuming. I can certainly relate to that. When I first began limiting the amount of fat I ate, I began to notice how much better I felt. As I began to lose weight, I began to feel even better. My energy level increased dramatically. I feel better today than I did when I was 20. Since I am 50, that is a pretty great feeling.

Not long ago my husband, Ken and I returned to that same mountain trail. This time I hiked every step of the way with him. A major storm had recently uprooted numerous trees on the trail and one blocked it entirely except for a little crawl space formed by some limbs that held it slightly off the ground. As I crawled on my hands and knees under that tree I thought to myself, "You know, Vicki, you were smarter when you sat in the car for 6 hours!"

I am still not crazy about hiking or any other kind of intense physical exertion. But it is such a thrill to know that I can do it. To me, the biggest benefit of having more energy is felt in more subtle ways. The fact that I can now exercise without agony and get through my daily routine with energy to spare is more important to me than being able to scale a tall mountain or do cartwheels. I am no longer a prisoner of my weight.

Let A Reader Inspire You

I have had the good fortune to hear terrific news from so many people who tell me that my recipes and tips have worked for them. A wonderful young woman named Selina Nobles has graciously allowed me to share several of the letters she has written to me with you. I think you will find them just as inspiring and motivating as I do.

Dear Mrs. Park,
I want to tell you what an answer to my prayers your cookbook has been to me. I have been overweight most of my life and have probably lost several thousand pounds and have gained twice that much back. Several months ago I became more depressed than I have ever been about my weight. I began to pray every night for God to fix whatever was wrong with my body that made me totally incapable of eating normally. He didn't heal my body but instead sent me your book. I have lost 42 pounds and my attitude about myself and my eating habits has completely changed.

I don't look at low-fat eating as a diet—it has simply become my way of life and I have made the adjustment so much easier that I have ever dreamed. Your book has given me a great basis for low-fat cooking and I am beginning to branch out on my own. I want you to know how much my attitude has changed about myself and my life. Even after only a 42 pound loss and knowing I have much more to go, I have made a start and am doing something about my weight instead of watching it just creep up. I feel so much better about myself that I almost can't imagine how I will feel when I reach my goal.

In the past, after losing weight I have always gained it back because I was never able to make the distinction between a diet and changing my eating habits. I have no fear about gaining weight back because, as I said, low-fat is simply the way I eat now. Thank you so much for *Live! Don't Diet!* It is making it possible for me to have my life back.

Sincerely,

Selina Nobles

Dear Mrs. Park,

As of last Thursday my total loss is exactly 80 pounds. Up to this point being a normal size has been a distant and intangible dream. For the first time in years, it is now a tangible reality. There is simply no way I can express my gratitude.

Love,

Selina

Hi Vicki!

I have now lost 103 pounds! I can't believe how my life has changed because of this weight loss. I have started wearing the most incredible clothes. I am going skydiving! Words cannot describe how incredible this change in my life is.

Love you so much,

Selina

Thank you, Selina, for your beautiful letters. I believe they convey so well the real joy we feel when we lose weight we need to lose, whether it is one pound or one hundred.

Section Two
A Lot Of Information

Let's Get Down To Basics

I promised you a little inspiration and a lot of information. Now that I've shared some things with you that I hope will motivate and inspire you, let's move on to the information I want to share.

But first, I have another corny joke. Well, it's kind of a joke. It has been a few pages since I have told one so get ready to groan again. It seems that two women were in their local pharmacy looking at the display of weight loss products. One of the women picked up a huge bottle of diet pills. As she read the list of ingredients she remarked to her companion, "I think I'll ask the pharmacist which is the very worst diet pill to take." "Don't bother", said the other woman. "I can answer that. The very worst diet pill to take is a friend who has lost a little weight and wants to tell you about it *over and over and over.*"

I won't do that, I promise. I'm just here to share the information that helped me lose. I'm a counselor by profession and a person who loves to share helpful information with people by nature. This carries over into all parts of my life. If I find a good sale, I'll call everyone I know and tell them about it. My mother often teases me by saying that I should have become a professional shopping consultant.

Well, back to business. First we'll talk about the basics, then we'll get to the tasty and simple low-fat recipes for everything from appetizers to desserts. In this section, the information I want to share will carry you through all aspects of healthier living the low-fat way—from weight loss and exercise information to how to cook, shop and plan low-fat menus. As with most things in life, there are basic guidelines you need to follow to be successful and that's what you'll find in this section. If you have read *Live! Don't Diet!* you may remember a few of these basics, which I also discussed there. However, they are so important that I can't repeat them enough. In addition, this book goes into much greater detail.

I recently heard the term "microwave mentality" used to describe people who want everything quick and easy. I love that expression. While it is probably meant to be derogatory, it fits me in many ways. I have a lot to do besides spending much of my time in the kitchen. Even though I love to eat, I want something that doesn't take hours to prepare. That is why I am so happy with my low-fat lifestyle.

As you read about the basics of low-fat living that you will find here, I think one thing will be quite clear. This way of eating and living is simple. There are not a lot of rules to follow or complicated menus to plan. Grocery shopping and cooking are easier than ever—and so is clean up. All of this would be worth changing to a low-fat lifestyle even if it did not have the wonderful benefits of potential weight loss and better health! So, come on, let's get down to basics.

The Basics Of Low-Fat Weight Loss

As my husband Ken and I watched the Super Bowl last year, the TV camera zoomed in on a huge defensive tackle who appeared to be perfectly square. He seemed at least 6' tall and 6' wide. The announcer, in relating the player's vital statistics, mentioned that he weighed 250 pounds. Ken and I together had lost more than that huge football player weighed! Then I thought about my own 180 pound loss. I realized that I had lost more than most average adult men weigh. I pictured myself bodily picking up a 180 pound man and trying to carry him. I couldn't do it. As a matter of fact, I probably couldn't even pick him up, much less carry him one step. Yet, my body was hauling around that much extra weight for much of my life. I can't believe I didn't keel over years ago.

You may need to lose only a few pounds but think of those pounds in terms of a 10 pound baby or a 40 pound toddler. Most of us have had to carry a sleeping child at one time or another. As much as we love the little darlings, after a few minutes they do get heavy. After a little while, our bodies start protesting with lower back aches, muscle strain and heavy breathing. At least we can put the child down. We can't just put the extra weight down. We have to carry it around endlessly unless we make the decision to do something about it.

Many of us have made that decision to do something about it many times—in my case about 10,000 times. Unfortunately, for the first 9,999 times I tried it the hard way. I tried every diet that came along. I would lose 5 pounds, then gain back 10 pounds. My biggest mistake was thinking about weight loss in terms of DIETING. This is a major blunder that most of us make. We go on a diet, lose the weight and then return to our old life-styles. Unfortunately, due to the "rabbit food" mentality of many diets, we never even make it to our goal weight. Even if we do, the lost weight returns rapidly once we return to our old eating habits.

It is so important to get rid of the idea of dieting. I cannot stress this strongly enough. The word in itself implies a short-term commitment. No one ever goes on a diet with the intention of remaining on it forever. What we must do is commit ourselves to a lifestyle change to healthier eating. While our main goal may be weight loss, it is best not to even think of it at all. Once you begin eating healthier, the excess weight will often naturally disappear.

Years ago a co-worker of mine was told to eat healthier by her doctor because of cholesterol problems. At lunch time, as I happily waddled off to a high-fat feast, I would always say to her, "Well, Sue, which pasture are you going to graze in today?" I, like many people, thought that healthy eating was condemnation to a lifetime of nothing but fodder. How wrong I was!

Healthy eating is nothing but making simple adjustments to the things we love to eat. I am still able to enjoy all the delicious dishes I have always loved, but now that I have learned to prepare them in a healthy way, I can enjoy them without guilt or fear.

While I am neither a nutritionist or a physician, I have used the wonderful things they learned and shared with the world to lose the weight I could never lose before. Here is what I learned that helped Ken and me finally lose weight and keep it off for more than five years now:

- I had heard that medical experts felt that lowering the fat in our food intake could not only improve health in many cases but could also help in weight loss. I talked to my own doctor and also began reading books from my local bookstore and library on low-fat weight loss. Most experts seemed to feel that keeping the fat intake in the 20-40 fat gram per day range is best for women who wish to lose and in the 30-50 gram range per day for men. I personally decided to keep my own intake in the 25-35 grams per day range. Anyone who is interested in lowering the amount of fat intake should talk to their physician or nutritionist to determine the range that is best for them and should also try to read what the experts say. There are loads of good books on the subject.

- After determining that I would try eating less fat, I purchased several small paperback books that give the fat content in most foods, including those served in chain restaurants. By purchasing several, I was able to keep one at home, at work and in my car. I began reading through them to educate myself on the fat content of my favorite foods. There were some surprises. I was happy to learn that some of the foods that I figured had loads of fat were really not so bad. Of course, the reverse was sometimes true!

- I began reading labels. Almost every packaged food sold commercially has a label that gives the nutritional analysis of the food. I paid particular attention to the number of fat grams per serving.

- I went through my kitchen and removed all the high-fat foods that I knew my family shouldn't eat and replaced them with their low-fat and fat-free equivalents. I resolved that I would simply enjoy these products for their own good taste and not make the mistake of comparing them to the high-fat product they replaced. Making that comparison is self-defeating. So what if the fat-free version doesn't taste quite as rich as the old high-fat original! I'm just grateful that I can enjoy lower-fat and no-fat versions of everything from sour cream to potato chips without guilt and without the fear that all that fat will someday kill me.

- I took all of my favorite recipes and began working on them to remove as much fat as possible while keeping all of the good taste. In most cases it was simply a matter of using a leaner cut of meat, a low-fat equivalent of a high-fat ingredient or a little extra spice.

- I resolved that I would not count calories. Calorie counting is too reminiscent of the old dieting mentality. I simply decided to eat until I was comfortably full. Eating lots of fiber-rich foods is a good way to get full and stay that way. Beans, grains and vegetables are especially filling.

- I tried to reduce my sugar intake as much as possible, because sugar makes me hungry. I'm not the only one. A friend of mine won't even chew regular chewing gum because the sugar in it makes her hungry. It is self-defeating to fill up on a delicious low-fat meal then make myself hungry all over again with a sugary dessert. I learned to make sugar-free and fat-free desserts and to eat commercially prepared fat-free cookies and cakes only sparingly since they are still often high in sugar.

- I trained myself to wait a few minutes before helping myself to seconds at mealtime. Often we don't realize how full we are until we stop eating for a moment.

- I determined that I would forever forget the word diet. I also resolved to not think about the fact that I was making any sort of "change" in my lifestyle. After all I was in my forties and pretty set in my ways. The idea of change didn't really appeal to me. I wanted to lose weight but I didn't want to have to change my life much to do it! I simply began using my low-fat and fat-free ingredients to prepare the dishes I had always prepared and always will prepare. It was simply a matter of using the healthier ingredients I now had on hand to make the dishes I loved. Because it is so painless, it has been so easy for me to maintain my healthier life and my weight loss. I know that I can prepare a low fat version of practically any dish that I want to eat.

A friend of mine, who lost 70 pounds through low-fat eating recently said to me, "Vicki, wouldn't it have been wonderful if doctors had learned about low-fat weight loss years ago. Just think of the heartache, the frustration and the years of letting fat ruin our lives that we could have been spared." Yes, it would have been wonderful, but I am just glad that they learned about it before I killed myself with fat.

The Basics Of Exercise

When I weighed 315 pounds, my attitude toward exercise was rather like that of my young relative. As a small child, he was, like me, a classic couch potato. His greatest form of exercise was pressing the buttons on the TV remote control. One day his father was particularly disturbed because he wanted to watch TV while the other children were playing ball. "Son," his dad exclaimed, "We are definitely going to have to get you on a good exercise program!" "Yipee!" the little boy replied. "I'm going to be on TV!"

I can relate to that. When I weighed 315 pounds I never did anything that required more than necessary movement if I could help it. As the old joke goes, the only exercise I ever got was pushing my luck! When I started eating healthy, I felt that if I also tried to begin an exercise program, I would be changing my lifestyle too much at once and would probably quickly quit. Therefore, I put exercising off. I didn't do any real exercise until I had lost over 100 pounds. I am not proud of that fact but in my case change had to come just a little at a time. I now realize I should have started exercising sooner.

We've already talked about making changes gradually. I started my healthier lifestyle by first changing the way I cooked. Then, in time came an exercise video with some easy walking movements. Now I have added workouts on a recumbent exercise bicycle and a treadmill to my routine. I try to do about 30-45 total minutes of exercise at least every other day. By taking little baby steps toward healthy eating and a healthy exercise program, I have been able to build up to a lifestyle that I would have quit in a heartbeat if I had started it all at once. I admit I should have started sooner but at least I finally got my act together. I am still no great fan of exercise but I do it because I know what it can do. Regular exercise can not only help us lose weight and keep it off, it can also help the body fight disease and reduce stress. Experts now say that it can possibly even extend your life. It's kind of like saving money. You might hate to do it, but the end results sure are nice.

Aerobic exercise is the most effective way to strengthen the heart and also contributes to both losing weight and keeping it off. There are excellent aerobic exercises for every taste and age. Brisk walking, either outdoors or on a treadmill, is an excellent aerobic exercise, as is cycling, running, jogging and stair climbing. Which ever exercise you choose, start slowly and build up. If you plan to buy exercise equipment such as a treadmill, stationary bicycle, stair climber or ski machine, spend some time trying them out in a store or health club before buying. Also question other people about their experiences with home exercise equipment. I bought my recumbent bicycle after a friend told me about hers. When she told me that it allows her to sit back in a comfortable seat and read while cycling, I knew I had to have one. That is definitely my kind of exercise!

For an inexpensive source of help in exercising, you may want to invest a few dollars in an exercise video. They range from very gentle workouts to really strenuous routines. A good way to find one that is right for you is to check out the selection at your local library or video rental store. You can try out the ones that seem right for you before buying.

Even the simple routines of daily life can be turned into effective exercise. Instead of casually strolling down the mall or to the mailbox, pick up your step and get some exercise out of it. If you work at a desk, get up and briskly walk around the office as frequently as possible. No matter what you are doing, put some pep into it and you will get the benefits of exercising your body.

Strength training is also important. Those exercises that tone the abdominals and other muscle groups aren't just for firming up, they are also helpful in giving muscles strength to protect us from some types of injury. No matter what kinds of exercise you are considering, your own personal program should be planned by you and your physician. You should begin any change in eating habits or exercise only with the advice and consent of your doctor. Food and exercise needs can vary considerably depending on the individual. Your health care professional can help you decide the perfect plan for you.

The Basics Of Low-Fat Menu Planning

Planning meals is tough. If we prepare the same meals all of the time, our families often complain of eating the same old thing. If we get adventurous and serve new dishes, they want their familiar comfort foods back. The recipes and the menus in *Exceed The Feed Limit!* are for low-fat versions of old favorites and for new dishes that make use of ingredients that are popular with everyone. These are the dishes and the menus I prepared for my family while we were losing our weight and that I still prepare all of the time. Speaking of family, these are recipes that can be enjoyed by all members of the family. Everyone needs to eat healthier.

I freely admit to being a person who doesn't like to spend much time in the kitchen. I just don't have the time since I still work at the job I have held for years in addition to doing housework and writing cookbooks. Even if I had lots of time I wouldn't want to spend it in the kitchen. I love to eat but lots of cooking and kitchen clean-up just isn't for me. I'm not too crazy about grocery shopping either. That's why the recipes and menus you'll find here are for very quick and simple dishes containing common ingredients.

On the following pages are a few suggestions for breakfast, lunch and dinner. I hope you will find them helpful. Happy cooking!

What's For Breakfast???

I am often asked what I eat for breakfast. As a matter of fact, the only question I am asked more frequently is if I have had a facelift, since I formerly had three chins and now I have just one. The answer to that, in case you wondered, is no. I need one but I am a world class chicken! The skin has a marvelous elasticity. If it didn't, I would be kicking flab out of the way with every step. But back to the subject of breakfast. Before I began my low-fat lifestyle, I never ate breakfast at all. I just made up for it later in the day by consuming everything in sight. It was only when I began to eat healthy that I realized how important it is to eat breakfast. I once read that eating breakfast gets the metabolism going strong again after it has slowed down during sleep. That sounds reasonable to me. The morning meal also satisfies our appetites after a night of fasting. If we skip breakfast, it can be more than 16 hours between dinner and lunch the next day. We tend to go wild after that long without food.

Now I never miss breakfast. However, since I must be at my job by 8:00 A.M., I tend to eat the same easy things every work day and save the more elaborate morning meals for the weekend. The recipes for some of my favorite weekend breakfast treats are on the following pages. Listed below are some of my regular work day breakfasts:

- Oatmeal doctored with sugar substitute, fat-free liquid margarine and cinnamon. I sometimes add chopped peaches or raisins.

- Bagels, English muffins or several slices of toast with reduced calorie preserves and fat-free cream cheese or fat-free liquid margarine.

- Ready to eat fat-free, low-sugar cereal and sliced fruit.

- Commercially prepared low-fat toaster waffles or pancakes with liquid fat-free margarine and sugar-free maple syrup.

- Sweet roll taste-alikes or pancake taste-alikes (see recipe index).

- A sandwich made from several slices of 98% fat-free ham (deli-sliced) and fat-free Cheddar cheese on toast or an English muffin.

It is also important to drink something with every meal. At breakfast, I usually have fat-free, sugar-free hot chocolate or an orange-flavored, sugar-free beverage. This tastes a lot like orange juice and is vitamin enriched but has practically no calories. I love fruit juice, which is fat-free but quite high in calories. I am ashamed to say it but I would rather save my calories for things to eat, not things to drink!

Let's Do Lunch

Whether we are at home or at work, it is easy to have a low-fat, filling lunch. Since most of us are too busy to cook at lunch time, sandwiches, salads and soups are often quick and simple to prepare. They are staples for many of us, especially if we have to pack a lunch for ourselves, our spouses and our children to eat at work or school.

It is terrific that there is such a fantastic selection of low-fat and fat-free sandwich ingredients, salad dressings and soups in the grocery store these days. Thin-sliced deli-style meats such as ham and turkey paired with fat-free cheese on hearty whole-grain bread are a wonderful lunch time treat, especially when dressed with a spicy mustard. It is fun to haunt the condiments aisle in the market to look at some of the unique and delicious mustards that are now available. You can even doctor fat-free mayonnaise with herbs or spices to concoct your own gourmet sandwich spreads. One neat trick is to add low-fat or fat-free dry salad dressing mix to the mayo. This makes a wonderful sandwich spread, salad dressing or dip.

I love great big sandwiches and a good way to add bulk to them is by adding lots of lettuce, tomato or sprouts. If you haven't tried alfalfa sprouts on a sandwich, do it. They are available in most grocery stores and add a terrific taste. If you have to eat on the job, you still don't have to limit your choices to cold sandwiches. A friend of mine puts a couple of fat-free wieners in a thermos then covers them with hot, low-fat onion or chicken soup. At lunch, she eats the soup, then makes herself hot dogs with the wieners. She also buys the big bags of pre-chopped salad ingredients available in most grocery stores and often makes herself a big salad in a sealable plastic bag. She adds some deli-sliced ham or turkey, a little fat-free cheese and has herself a lovely chef's salad with just a few minutes work. Before adding the salad ingredients to the bag, she pours in her dressing. It remains at the bottom of the bag until lunch time, when she shakes the bag to distribute it. That way it doesn't wilt the greens. She eats from the bag, then throws it away. No empty bowl to have to take home!

Many offices provide microwave ovens for the use of their employees, which really opens up the possibilities for quick, hot lunches. From frozen commercially-prepared low-fat meals to leftovers from the night before, the microwave allows us to eat what we please. It also makes possible break time treats such as low-fat popcorn or even nachos.

I work in an office that provides a microwave and refrigerator for the use of employees, but to be honest, I seldom make use of them because I like to eat out at lunch. Most fast food and full service restaurants now provide low-fat menu selections that make it easy to dine out any time of day. Many chain restaurants even have pamphlets giving the nutritional information on all of their foods that are available if you ask. Some even print it on the menu. Of course, books listing the fat grams in foods also usually include chain restaurants. Even those restaurants that do not have low-fat menu items are usually very accommodating if you ask them to prepare your selection in a low-fat manner.

Some offices provide cafeterias for their employees. Many are very responsive to requests for low-fat selections. I was very honored when I was told that a group of employees gave a copy of my book *Live! Don't Diet!* to their cafeteria manager and requested that she prepare dishes from it. She now regularly offers low-fat selections and even posts the fat grams in the day's selections.

Just as with breakfast and dinner, you have complete freedom to choose delicious, low-fat hot or cold meals at lunch. You can enjoy a homemade treat or eat out without the least deprivation and with the knowledge that you are treating your body right! What could be easier or more gratifying?

The Age-Old Question:
What's For Dinner?

I imagine that thousands of years ago cave-dwelling cooks stood over their fires at the last minute and pondered what to fix for dinner, just as I do practically every night. I am the type person who never knows what I plan to serve until I get home from work and see what is in my refrigerator. Fortunately, most of my low-fat recipes are so easy they can be made in minutes.

For those of you who like to plan your meals, I have put together a few suggested menus from some of the recipes in this book. As for me, I'll probably still throw things together at the last minute. Organizational skills are one type of self-improvement that I'm too disorganized to ever learn! I'm the same way with cooking. I have good intentions about planning meals in advance but never get around to it.

I have read that the more dishes that are served as part of a meal, the more we tend to eat. That sounds like a perfect reason to prepare fewer dishes. I'm open to any justification for cooking less! That's why I usually serve just a main course with one or two vegetables or a salad.

Onion Baked Steak*
Fat-Free Mashed Potatoes*
Steamed Carrots

Chicken Picante*
Steamed Rice
Mexican Corn*

Steak In A Stew*
Delicious Layered Slaw*
Warm French Bread

Rich Ravioli Casserole*
Green Beans
Kind Of Greek Salad*

Quick And Tender Turkey*
My Favorite Sweet Potatoes*
English Peas

Lemon-Herb Chicken*
Easy Baked Rice*
Sautéed Broccoli*

Slow Cooker Oriental Beef*
Steamed Rice
Jellied Fresh Fruit Salad*

American Dinner Pie*
Snappy Cabbage*
Comforting Cornbread*

Hearty White Chili*
Crunchy Apple Salad*
Comforting Cornbread*

Crispy Oven Chicken*
Barbecued Potatoes*
Cole Slaw

Tasty Tamale Pie*
Mexican Spinach Salad*

Shortcut Lasagna*
Mixed Green Salad

Busy Day Ham And Dumplings*
Steamed Broccoli
Mixed Green Salad

Country-Style Pork*
Autumn Fruited Rice*
Squash Casserole*

*Denotes Recipes In This Book

The Basics Of Low-Fat Shopping

Before I wised up to the benefits of eating low-fat, my favorite meal was a big charcoal-broiled ribeye steak, a baked potato dripping with butter and a salad topped with loads of creamy dressing, followed by a huge piece of cheesecake. No wonder I weighed 315 pounds. Actually, I can still enjoy this meal and not have to worry about it. Now I eat a sensibly-sized sirloin with the visible fat removed and a large baked potato with fat-free liquid margarine and fat-free sour cream. My salad is still topped with creamy dressing and I still have cheesecake, although now the dressing and cheesecake are fat-free. This meal is just as good to me as the high-fat version used to be because I know I can have it without harming my health or my weight.

There are those among you who may be saying, "The low-fat versions just aren't as tasty! I'll never be able to get used to fat-free sour cream or cheese." Don't let yourself think this way. It is terribly self-defeating. Those low-fat versions of my favorite high-fat foods enabled me to continue eating my favorite meals—the ones that caused me to weigh 315 pounds—while losing 180 pounds. I could still have cheesy lasagna, rich casseroles and creamy desserts. I didn't have to give them up for the rest of my life. I certainly believe the slight difference in taste is worth it! Besides, in a very short time the low-fat versions will begin to taste better to you than the high-fat ones.

If you think about it, fat has no taste. It just has an oily richness that acts as a conveyor of the flavors of the other ingredients in a dish. That's right! The flavors are in the other ingredients, not the fat. By giving up the fat you are not giving up flavor. You are only allowing yourself to enjoy the true, delicious taste of your foods.

It can truly become an adventure to go grocery shopping when you are living a low-fat lifestyle. Every day more and more great low-fat products are appearing on the shelves, thanks to the demand of health conscious consumers. I recently came home from grocery shopping and told my husband, "I have got to get a life! The most exciting thing that happened to me today was discovering a delicious new fat-free, 10 calorie per serving cheese spread at the store!" I was just kidding, but it really is fun to discover new products that we can enjoy. After all, much of life is centered around food. Just because we are living a healthy lifestyle doesn't mean we don't love to eat!

When you shop for groceries there are some things you definitely need to remember. I have said it before and will say it over and over—LEARN TO READ THE NUTRITIONAL DATA ON LABELS! Pay particular attention to the amount of fat in each serving. If you have special dietary needs, due to health problems, you may also need to monitor the sodium content and the saturated fat content. Even if you do not have special needs, you may wish to monitor the sodium content, particularly if you retain water easily.

While I don't count calories, I do pay attention to the calories per serving on labels. If one brand is lower in calories than another, I will buy that brand. I also try to avoid purchasing snacks and desserts that have a zillion calories per serving despite their low fat content because I know myself well enough to know that one serving of them is never enough for me. Consuming a half gallon of fat-free ice cream at 90 calories per half-cup will not help us lose weight!

On the following pages, I would like to share with you some of the ingredients that allowed me to lose 180 pounds and Ken to lose 90 pounds without deprivation. These are simply some of the basic foods that are important not only in losing weight, but in living a healthy lifestyle. As you live your own healthier lifestyle, you will discover more and more foods that you and your family can enjoy, but this may help you. Let's get out the grocery cart and get started!

Beef

Many people have the misconception that beef is loaded with fat but that isn't necessarily true. As with all meats, you simply have to eat the lower-fat cuts, remove all visible fat and cut back on portions. The difference in the amount of fat in the different cuts of beef can be astonishing. A 3-ounce serving of prime rib can have a whopping 30 grams of fat, while a 3-ounce serving of top round roast can have as few as 6 grams.

When buying beef, always buy top round or top sirloin, because those cuts are lowest in fat. Be sure to also remove any visible fat remaining. If buying ground beef, ask the butcher to freshly grind top round trimmed of all fat. In many grocery stores, ultra-lean ground beef is sold already packaged. Be sure that the amount of fat per serving is listed on the label and it is below 10 grams per serving. Many stores market specially pre-pared ground beef that has as little as 7 grams of fat per serving.

Since low-fat cuts of beef and low-fat ground beef do not have enough fat to keep them from sticking when sautéed, it is important to lightly spray your skillet with no-stick cooking spray. Low-fat cuts of beef may also be less tender, so you may wish to marinate them before cooking or sprinkle them with commercially prepared meat tenderizer.

If you are preparing ground beef for a casserole, soup or sauce, it is important to remove any fat remaining after cooking by blotting the meat with paper towels. You may also want to put the cooked ground beef in a colander and run hot water over it, then pat it dry. I have done this for a number of years now and have never had any problems with my plumbing result from it, but if you have delicate plumbing, you may need to skip this step.

If you are serving beef or any meat, learn to make it a sup-porting player in your meal, not the star attraction. Serve it with lots of vegetables on the side, or better still, make it part of a cas-serole, soup or pasta sauce. You will be surprised at how far a little meat will go when it is combined with other ingredients. Six ounces of meat, either ground or cut into small bite-sized pieces, will serve a whole family. You will still get a bit of meat in each bite. After all, it's the flavor and texture of the meat that counts. It doesn't take huge chunks of it. When I began cooking low-fat, I reduced the ground beef in my chili from 2 pounds to 6 ounces. I simply added more beans, onions and tomatoes to make up for it. It was actually better. I made similar adjustments in all of my recipes containing meat. I really got many more compliments from my family after I changed the recipes!

Pork

I never expected that pork could be part of a low-fat life-style, but we eat it regularly at my house. Like beef, pork can vary from very high in fat to very low in fat. Here again the important point is to read labels and make sure you are buying pork and pork products that are low in fat. Pork tenderloin, trimmed of all visible fat, contains only 4 fat grams in a 3-ounce serving. On the other hand, spareribs can contain 26 grams of fat in 3 ounces and pork shoulder can contain 13 grams in the same size serving. Since I only want to use the cut that is lowest in fat, I always buy tenderloin. It can be roasted whole, sliced into chops or cutlets, cubed for kebobs and stews or cut into thin slivers for stir-frying. I even slice it into long strips to barbecue like spareribs on occasion

More low-fat and no-fat pork products are becoming available every day. It is possible to buy ham and wieners that have practically no fat, as well as low-fat smoked sausage. Fat-free cold cuts, such as salami and bologna are also available. We have hot dogs and ham sandwiches at our house regularly. Along with the low-fat dairy products, the growing availability of low-fat meats has made it so easy to eat like a normal person. We don't have to sacrifice a thing!

Poultry

Surprisingly, chicken and turkey breast are similar in fat content to the leanest cuts of beef and pork. That may especially interest the people who think that they can only eat chicken if they are eating low-fat. However, it is good to serve chicken and turkey often, since they can be prepared in so many terrific ways. In fact, many recipes featuring pork can be used interchangeably with those containing chicken or turkey.

It is best to use only the breast meat of chicken or turkey since it is considerably lower in fat than the dark meat. A 3-ounce portion of breast meat contains about 3 fat grams. Never eat the skin. There is a lot of fat in poultry skin. Many food experts do feel that it doesn't matter whether the skin is removed before or after cooking.

I usually buy boneless, skinless chicken breasts since they are quick and easy to work with, but the bone-in breasts work equally well in most recipes. The availability of turkey cutlets and boneless roasts cut from the breast also makes regularly serving turkey so easy. It is not just a holiday treat anymore.

If you are buying a fresh or frozen turkey or turkey breast, be sure to notice if the label states whether or not it has been pre-basted. Some turkeys are injected with oil to make the meat more moist. Others are injected with broth. The solution used to baste the turkey may raise the fat content of the meat considerably. Choose only those that have been pre-basted with broth or with nothing.

Ground turkey is another product we need to purchase selectively. Some people like to use it in place of ground beef. Make sure the ground turkey you buy is 100% breast meat only. Some ground turkey even contains skin and is high in fat. If you cannot find 100% pure ground turkey breast, have the butcher grind it for you.

Precooked, low-fat turkey breast pieces and ham pieces, weighing 1-2 pounds are available in most grocery stores, as are precooked chicken breasts. Since I like to spend as little time in the kitchen as possible, I keep these on hand to use in casseroles and stir-fried dishes, as well as in sandwiches. Using precooked turkey and chicken breasts can cut down considerably on time when you don't want to have to cook the meat from scratch. If you must be careful about sodium, look for low-sodium brands, since processed meats are often quite high in sodium. Speaking of processed meats, both turkey and chicken-based low-fat versions of popular sandwich meats such as ham, salami, bologna and wieners are on the market.

Chicken and turkey are not only delicious hot, they are equally good cold. After all, who doesn't love a wonderful chicken salad or sliced turkey sandwich? For versatility and taste, chicken and turkey are a terrific part of a healthy and wonderful low-fat lifestyle.

Seafood

Remember this corny joke: "I'm on the seafood diet—I eat all the food I see!" I can relate to that, even if it is a joke. In years gone by that was the only diet I could ever stick to! Well, all joking aside, seafood can be a wonderful addition to our low-fat menus. As always, you need to read labels carefully since some types of fish are much higher in fat that others. Cod, flounder, grouper, haddock, perch, pike, pollock and snapper only average 1 gram of fat in a 3-ounce serving while mackerel can contain up to 12 grams.

Practically all varieties of shellfish are very low in fat. Lobster, crabs and scallops have only 1 gram in a 3-ounce serving, while shrimp, oysters and mussels have as many as 2 grams per serving. Since fish or seafood is especially delicious grilled, sautéed or steamed, it is easy to prepare ultra low-fat seafood main dishes. However, even that old favorite, fried seafood can be made in a delicious low-fat way by using our oven-frying technique or by frying it in only 1 tablespoon of oil.

If you think the old days of drawn butter or tartar sauce served along with your favorite seafood are behind you if you are eating low-fat, think again. Liquid fat-free margarine with a little lemon makes a terrific drawn butter-style dipping sauce, while delicious fat-free tartar sauce is available in stores. It can also be made at home.

Many grocery stores now feature fresh seafood counters. They have every kind of fresh fish and shellfish you can imagine. Not only do they sell great seafood, they will tell you the best ways to prepare it and may even steam it for you if you ask. My grocery store's seafood counter features a section of special spices, seasonings and sauces to use in preparing fish and shell-fish. Some of the special seasonings are even good on vegetables or in dips or salad dressings. As I like to say—experiment!

Cheeses

Hooray for the makers of fat-free and low-fat cheeses! From fat-free cottage cheese in rich lasagna to fat-free cream cheese in silky cheesecake to fat-free Cheddar in gooey casseroles, these wonderful products are among the most important because they enable us to enjoy so many dishes that were previously taboo to those wanting to lose weight or eat healthy. After all, many cheeses have a tremendous 9 fat grams per ounce—and who can eat just one ounce?

Some years ago, I bought a package of fat-free shredded Cheddar cheese at the grocery. As the cashier totaled my purchases, she picked up the package of cheese and said "Is this stuff any good?" "Yes, if you like to eat pencil erasers," I replied, only half in jest. At the time I didn't know how to use it properly. Many people still don't, which is one reason they sometimes complain that they don't like it.

With the exception of fat-free Parmesan cheese, many types of fat-free cheese do not come out well when used to top a casserole or dish that requires lengthy cooking. They get hard. It is best to add these cheeses just before serving and let the heat of the dish melt them. Briefly topping the dish with a piece of foil or plastic wrap can hold in the heat and help the melting process. Shredded fat-free cheese works best when it is layered or mixed with other ingredients in a casserole. Then it acts and tastes much like regular shredded Cheddar.

Some people I know like to have the best of both worlds. They will use fat-free shredded cheese in a casserole, but will use a tablespoon or two of finely shredded regular cheese as a topping or in combination with the fat-free cheese. When divided between 4 servings of a casserole or other entree, this only adds a few fat grams, so you might like to try doing this yourself.

Today, you can find a fat-free version of almost any cheese from cream cheese to mozzarella. If you haven't tried fat-free cheese recently, I suggest you try it again. Many of them are now quite delicious. Some of the processed fat-free cheeses are especially good and melt really well. Try several brands. You may find you like one better than another. If you plan to eat a fat-free cheese in a salad or sandwich or with crackers, I suggest you let it come to room temperature first. This enhances the flavor and texture.

Personally, I am eternally grateful to the makers of fat-free cheese. So what if it isn't always quite as rich and delicious as the high-fat version. I have grown to love it because it allows me to enjoy many of my very favorite dishes without fat or fear.

Sour Cream

Creamy dips, gooey casseroles, rich sauces. Where would these treats be without sour cream? At 45 fat grams per cup, sour cream is both the curse and the blessing of many wonderful dishes. That is why it is so terrific that we can enjoy sour cream and all of the dishes it so wonderfully enhances without the fat. Fat-free sour cream is a real boon to the weight and health conscious.

Once I made plain old California dip with fat-free sour cream and dehydrated onion soup mix, which also has no fat. I took it to a social gathering, along with fat-free chips. I thought I had made enough for a huge crowd but it was gone in minutes.

People could not get enough of it. Two small children ate about a pint each before their Mom pulled them away. This not only shows the great taste of fat-free foods but also how readily children will eat them. Only small babies need much fat in their diet. If we begin to train our children to enjoy low-fat foods early in life, they will no doubt lead healthier lives.

Fat-free sour cream is an especially welcome product because it can replace some of the creaminess and rich taste that fat used to add to our foods. For example, I use fat-free sour cream instead of butter and whole milk in preparing packaged macaroni and cheese. Like many packaged mixes, the macaroni and cheese contains very little fat until you add the butter and whole milk at home. The sour cream is a great replacement.

Eggs And Egg Substitutes

A medium egg contains 5 fat grams. Practically all of the fat is in the yolk. While nutritionists recommend limiting eggs to three per week, people with high cholesterol may need to limit them even further, depending upon the advice of their physician or nutritionist. While it is best to eat high-fiber fruits and breads or whole-grain cereals for breakfast, if you feel that you must eat eggs, try scrambling several egg whites with a little yellow food color added. That way you can enjoy eggs without any fat. Use no-stick cooking spray to keep the eggs from sticking. Serve with several low-fat ham slices or low-fat smoked sausage and toast. If you enjoy stuffed eggs for lunches or picnics, try stuffing the cooked whites with seasoned fat-free cream cheese, chicken salad or tuna salad.

Fat-free egg substitutes are a terrific way to enjoy eggs without the fat and without the trouble of separating the white from the yolk. Egg substitutes are ready to use right out of the carton. If you hate to clean up, that means no shells to have to throw away or extra bowls to wash. If you use egg substitutes exclusively, that also means having more room in the refrigerator since there are no large egg cartons taking up space.

"But I want real eggs!" you may be saying. Most egg substitutes are real eggs. They are made from egg whites. They are indistinguishable from whole eggs when used to prepare baked goods. They also make very tasty scrambled eggs and omelets. As an added bonus, most brands have only 30-40 calories per ¼ cup serving compared to 79 in a whole egg. Try several brands to find the one you like best.

Oils, Cooking Sprays And Margarine

There is no way around it, cooking oils are pure fat and have an average 12-14 fat grams per tablespoon. That makes their use limited on a low-fat lifestyle, unless you want to blow all of your daily fat allowance on a few tablespoons of oil for frying. Not me. I want to use my fat grams for real food! If you must, you can prepare pan fried foods by cooking several servings with 1 tablespoon of oil. However, you can use no-stick cooking sprays to fry or sauté without any oil or butter. Just keep the heat fairly low. Better still, use the oven-frying technique that I use in several of the recipes in this book. Just lightly spray the pan with cooking spray, add the food, which is also lightly sprayed and bake at a medium-high temperature. Cooking sprays are available in a variety of flavors including butter-flavor and olive oil-flavor. Just remember that cooking sprays also contain oil and don't go overboard when using them. Most cooking sprays contain about 1 fat gram in a 1¼-second application. This is enough to coat a skillet or casserole dish.

When I began eating low-fat one of the things I missed most was butter and margarine. Butter and margarine have 11-12 fat grams per tablespoon. Even reduced-fat margarines contain an average 5 grams per tablespoon. Then, several years ago ultra-low fat and fat-free margarines began appearing on the shelves. That was a great day for me. While the original products took some getting used to, they are getting better and better. Some of the new fat-free liquid margerines are almost as tasty as the real thing and are almost calorie-free.

Milk

We have always been told how good milk is for us, yet a 1-cup serving of whole milk contains 8 fat grams. It also contains 150 calories. As the public becomes more health conscious, whole milk is becoming less popular. Since it is so high in fat, you can see why. Many consumers now use 2% milk instead. However 2% milk still contains 5 fat grams and has 121 calories in a 1-cup serving. Even 1% milk has 3 fat grams per cup. Why not have the pleasures of milk without any of the fat? Learn to use skim milk. Once you do, you won't know the difference. As a matter of fact, lots of people who have made the change say that even 1% milk now tastes unpleasantly oily to them and whole milk is like drinking cream.

Some brands of skim milk are better than others. Try them till you find the one you like best. Some of them are virtually indistinguishable from whole milk in appearance and are quite delicious. Adding a little non-fat dry milk powder or evaporated skim milk to the carton can make them even more like whole milk.

Non-fat dry milk and evaporated skim milk are also good to use in cooking when you want a richer milk flavor. They have no fat, yet can make cream sauces and other recipes containing milk seem almost decadently rich.

Buttermilk is also a terrific way to add great flavor to foods. Despite its name, low-fat buttermilk is commonly available. It can also perk up a variety of foods, from soups to salad dressings. If you don't use a lot of buttermilk, you might prefer powdered low-fat buttermilk.

Mayonnaise And Salad Dressing

In the past, the most complaints I heard about the taste of a low-fat food was about mayonnaise. Practically everybody hated it. In truth, it used to taste a lot like wallpaper paste must taste—gummy and bland. But as with many low-fat and fat-free versions of our favorite high-fat foods, the quality has improved dramatically.

Quite frankly, I didn't use fat-free mayonnaise for a number of years, having tried it and found it terrible. I preferred instead to use fat-free Ranch salad dressing in recipes that called for mayonnaise. However, about a year ago I tried fat-free mayonnaise again and found it to be much better. I use it all the time now in all of the same ways I formerly used the high-fat version. It is fun to use it by the heaping spoonfuls without guilt.

I really don't know how we could ever be so crazy about real mayonnaise to start with. Not only does it have 11 fat grams and 100 calories in a tablespoon, but the primary ingredients are oil and eggs. That doesn't sound too appetizing, does it? Well, despite its drawbacks, it does taste wonderful and fortunately the current fat-free versions come closer than ever to capturing its taste. If you still can't get used to it, try the next best thing, the reduced-fat version. You can find at least one national brand that has only 3 fat grams per tablespoon.

While low-fat and fat-free salad dressings have always been quite good, they also continue to improve in taste. Commercially prepared low-fat and fat-free dressings are available bottled and as dried packaged mixes that you prepare at home. The dried mixes are really versatile. They can be added to fat-free mayonnaise to make a great dip or sandwich spread.

Cereals

Cereals are a vital part of healthy eating—and not just at breakfast. Cereal makes a really great snack too. As with most foods, there are some really healthy cereals and some really unhealthy ones. It is important to shop carefully. A number of cereals are fairly low in fat but still high in sugar. Try to avoid these. Choose cereals that are not only low in fat but low in sugar or sugar-free.

If you are really interested in eating healthy, some of the no-frills cereals are the best choices. Basic cereals, such as shredded wheat and bran-based cereals are full of fiber and nutrients. As we know, fiber is vital to good health and also helps us keep that full feeling that is so important when we are trying to lose weight.

In addition to being so good for us, the basic cereals have another benefit. They are usually less expensive than the cereals that have added fruits or other frills. They are also easier to find in generic brands, which can help cut costs even further. If you want fruit, you can add it yourself at home. You can even flavor plain cereal up with some spices. A little cinnamon or nutmeg, along with a sprinkle of granulated sugar substitute can made a basic cereal seem more special. At our house, cereal often substitutes for a snack or dessert.

When buying cereals, don't pass the hot cereals up. They are also an extremely important addition to a low-fat lifestyle. Not only are they healthful, they are a real comfort food. Nothing is more satisfying that starting or ending the day with a big bowl of hot cereal. I love to dress it up with fruit, cinnamon, granulated sugar substitute and fat-free liquid margarine. My favorite hot cereal is oatmeal but I also love cream of wheat. When buying oatmeal, get the quick-cooking variety rather than the instant kind that comes in packets. I personally find that the quick-cooking kind has a much more appealing texture than the instant since it retains more of the whole-grain consistency that makes it so good for you. Cream of wheat and multi-grain hot cereals are also great choices for a quick, warming start to a busy day.

Condiments

If vegetables, breads and grains are the heart of a low-fat lifestyle, condiments and spices are its soul. Consider this: when you season your foods with butter or oils, you are adding nothing but a greasy, slick taste. In contrast, condiments such as salsas, relishes, jams and preserves add sparkle and interest without any with Mexican food, or the marvelous pure fruit flavor of preserves spread on warm bread.

Check out all the various sections of your grocery where condiments are found. Don't forget the jam, jellies and syrups, the sauces and gravies, the pickles and relishes. An amazing number of them are fat-free or low-fat. It is fun to see just how many of these wonderful treats there are. Eating can never get dull!

While the stores are full of enough condiments to keep you happy forever, there is something very gratifying about making your own from time to time. Summer, when vegetables and fruits are plentiful and inexpensive, is the ideal time to treat yourself to homemade relishes or jams. They can be made in minutes and many of them can be successfully frozen or canned for later use.

I like to use aspartame-based sugar substitute in my homemade condiments instead of sugar. This removes a significant amount of calories. I am ashamed to say that I have been known to eat a whole jar of homemade preserves in one day. Since they contain nothing but fruit, sugar substitute and pectin, I can do it without feeling guilty. Of course, my family gets mad at me for eating them up, since they love them too.

I prefer to freeze homemade condiments made with sugar substitutes, when I make them in quantity. However, the makers of sugar substitutes and the makers of canning products are beginning to come out with recipes using sugar substitutes in canned goods. If you like to can your condiments, but don't want to use sugar, you might consult the recipe books put out by the major canning product makers.

While they are not technically considered condiments, herbs and spices also lend zest to your recipes. If fact, many food experts say that adding them to your food is an ideal way to make up for the fat you have taken out. The spice section of the grocery is full of familiar and not so familiar spices, as well as other marvelous flavoring agents, including extracts and seasoning blends.

Remember to also check out the produce section. Fresh herbs are often available in season.

There are a million ways to use condiments and spices to add thrill to your meals. A spoonful of relish is terrific with dried beans or sliced ham. It can also be added to fat-free mayonnaise to make a spicy salad dressing. Spicy salsas are turning up in everything from main dishes to dips. Jams and jellies are not just for breakfast anymore. They are finding their way into everything from appetizers to desserts.

While fancy restaurants wouldn't be caught dead with a ketchup bottle on the table, many neighborhood eateries keep an array of condiments on every table. The restaurants do it to save the server steps. Since I am generally the server in my house, I like to save steps too. I keep everyday condiments that aren't refrigerated, like mustard, ketchup, steak sauce and hot sauce in a little basket in my cupboard. That way they can be whisked out at mealtime.

Whether you prefer the comforting flavors of these everyday condiments or the more exotic tastes of condiments from around the world, they make your low-fat lifestyle an adventure. That is definitely not the case with dull old butter or oil. Now, aren't you glad they are out of your life!

Breads

I have always loved bread. When I was a very chubby child, my Mom would try in vain to keep me from pigging out. Once, as I stuffed another roll in my mouth, Mom said reprovingly, "Vicki, three rolls!" "No, Mom," I said, patting my fat little tummy, "just one great big roll." As I grew older that one great big roll that was my stomach did grow into three, or maybe four. Amazing as it may be, bread helped me lose that tummy and go from a size 52 to size 8.

Most breads are surprisingly low in fat. They are also very filling and very comforting. With the exception of croissants and some specialty breads, even most commercially prepared breads have little more than ½ to 1 gram of fat per slice. However, as always, be sure to read the nutritional information on the package before purchasing. It is best to eat whole-grain breads. The dense, chewy texture of whole grain breads makes them especially satisfying, as well as more nutritious. If you would like two slices of bread for the calorie cost of one, you'll want to try the reduced-calorie breads. It is also possible to buy reduced-calorie buns and rolls. Most breads are great served plain, but a little fat-free or low-fat margarine or low-sugar jam can make them extra-special.

While most of us may be too busy to prepare time-consuming homemade breads, even making a simple quick bread from scratch can give you a great sense of satisfaction, a delicious treat to eat, and, as an added bonus, a heavenly aroma coming from your kitchen! Even if you have just a minute, you can make fresh bread for your family.

One of the most popular members of the bread family is the bagel. Once a specialty of the big city, every crossroads now has a shop where fresh bagels are prepared daily. Even convenience stores have a supply in their freezer. Since they are extremely low in fat and very filling, they are great for healthy eating. But beware. Some of them can contain over 400 calories each—so don't get carried away!

English muffins are also wonderful. Like bagels, they now come in every flavor under the sun and can provide a great breakfast or snack. English muffins and bagels are also really versatile. Whether you eat them plain, use them for sandwiches or for instant pizza, they can add heartiness and terrific taste to our low-fat menus.

To round out our shopping tour of the bread department, don't forget the tortillas. In many stores it is possible to find packaged fresh tortillas. The taste of the fresh tortillas is especially wonderful. If you have the time one day, you might even like to try making your own. They are not difficult and are worth the effort. Both corn and flour tortillas are really jacks of all trades. Serve either along with your main course just as you would any bread.

Corn tortillas, of course, are also essential for such wonderful treats as tacos and enchiladas They can also be used to make homemade tortilla chips. Flour tortillas are just as versatile. They can be used for a multitude of purposes from burritos to dumplings. A dampened flour tortilla pressed into a pie plate can even pinch-hit for pie crust. While fat-free corn and flour tortillas are available, most regular tortillas are still very low in fat. Tortillas can also be found in both the refrigerated and frozen foods section of your grocery store.

Vegetables, Fruits And Grains

When I was a child my Mom would tease me about being a "bottomless pit" because she could never fill me up. I just loved to eat. That is how I eventually ended up weighing 315 pounds. Well, I'm guess I'm still a bottomless pit. I still love to eat. The big difference is that I have learned what to eat. I used to fill up on junk food. I still fill up on things that taste good but the big difference is that these things are also good for me. Vegetables, fruits and grains are by far the most essential foods to those of us who want to lose weight and eat healthy. They are not only nutritious but are also very filling. They are, for the most part, fiber-rich and foods that are high in fiber keep us satisfied. Because I fill up on them, I'm not tempted to fall off the wagon.

Fresh vegetables and fruits are no longer just seasonal treats. During our winter, they are imported from countries south of the equator where it is the summer growing season. On the iciest days we can have fresh asparagus, watermelon and strawberries as well as exotic fruits and vegetables that are totally new to us. It is fun to buy new vegetables and fruits which may be unfamiliar and experiment with them.

With the availability of the microwave oven and electronic steamers, fresh vegetable preparation has never been easier. Some stores even package them already trimmed, cleaned and ready for cooking. Frozen vegetables and unsweetened frozen fruits are also convenient options. The ultimate in convenience is canned vegetables and fruits. Try to buy low-sodium canned vegetables or rinse them well since they are often high in sodium. Always buy juice-packed canned fruits rather than those in sugar-sweetened syrup.

While all vegetables are mega-important, some, such as beans, potatoes, brown rice and other whole grains are particularly vital. They are "power foods"—high in satisfying carbohydrates and fiber, yet extremely low in fat. "But pigging out on a potato just isn't as much fun as pigging out on chocolate cake!" you may be saying. Nonsense! What does pigging out on chocolate cake get you except fatter and more depressed? You can eat a whole pound of tasty oven-fried, fat-free French fries for less calories than a little piece of chocolate cake. A pound of French fries is not only fun but will fill you up and keep you full. The cake won't do anything but make you want more. Which would you rather be—full, fit and fabulous or just plain fatter by the day? The foods you feed yourself will make all the difference.

Seasoning is very important in making our vegetables taste special without fat. The new liquid fat-free margarines are wonderful on vegetables and a little low-fat deli-sliced ham adds a delightful smoky taste to green vegetables and dried beans.

Chicken bouillon is also great to season many vegetables. Don't forget gravy! Make your own fat-free gravy with flour, beef or chicken bouillon and skim milk or water. I usually opt for the commercially prepared gravies from the grocery. Many are very low in fat.

Load up your shopping cart with as many vegetables, fruits and grains as your refrigerator or cupboard will hold. With the exception of the avocado, they are all virtually fat-free. Make them the sun around which your low-fat world revolves. You may be rewarded with better health, more energy and the figure of your dreams!

Desserts

Desserts can be the most wonderful and the most terrible things in the world. Like a really gorgeous person who is terribly shallow, desserts look magnificent while hiding the fact that they often have no nutritional value. In fact, they could also be compared to a really gorgeous person who is also a hit-man since they might eventually kill you if you aren't careful. Okay, maybe I'm being overly dramatic but you know what I mean. They are too often loaded with fat and sugar, which over time can lead your body into deep trouble.

Since I am a sugar addict, I try to make desserts that are totally sugar-free or very low in sugar. As I have mentioned before, a little sugar just makes me want more. Even if cookies, ice cream or cake are fat-free, they can be loaded with tons of empty sugar calories. As much as we would like to think otherwise, you can't eat unlimited amounts of that stuff and lose weight. While fat-free and sugar free ice cream can still carry quite a caloric wallop if eaten in unlimited amounts, some of the aspartame-sweetened fruit flavored popsicles now on the market contain as little as 15 calories each. You could eat a whole box of these in one day and not be in much trouble.

The ideal solution is to eat desserts that are fat-free and sweetened with sugar substitute, even though we still need to limit these to sensible amounts. Sugar-free, fat-free puddings and gelatins can be used to make a variety of delicious desserts, as can fresh and canned fruits. Speaking of fruit, don't ignore fresh fruit as a dessert or snack. It is more filling than pudding, pie or cake and is more nutritionally valuable as well. A melange of fruit and melon chunks makes a most attractive and delicious dessert, even for company. One of the most memorable desserts I ever had was a gorgeous assortment of fresh mixed fruits served in a stemmed goblet and topped at the last minute with sparkling club soda. Create beautiful, healthy desserts and congratulate yourself on being both gorgeous and intelligent!

The Basics Of Low-Fat Cooking

My daughter, Ashley likes to joke that I should have named my first book *Live! Don't Fry It!* instead of *Live! Don't Diet!* While I have to give her points for that one, it isn't quite true. You can still enjoy the crisp taste of fried foods when you are eating low-fat. It's just that you fry them in a healthier way. Almost any method of cooking can be used to prepare low-fat treats but some of the most delightful and familiar flavors can be created by oven-frying and sautéing since many of our favorite comfort foods before we started watching our fat intake were fried.

Microwaving and steaming are also great ways to enjoy the delicious taste of vegetables with little time or trouble. On the next few pages, I would like to share with you the basics of these tried and true cooking techniques.

"Frying" The Low-Fat Way

Some time in the very, very distant future, anthropologists will be digging around in the relics of our era and will come across one of our cookbooks. They will be mystified by the fact that the seemingly intelligent and sophisticated people of our day actually cooked food by throwing it into a vat of boiling fat until it was brown and hard. This (along with trying to figure out the purpose of a man's necktie!) will completely baffle them. Actually it is already starting to baffle many people here and now. Frying not only completely hides the natural taste of the food, it is unhealthy and messy. That last reason alone is reason enough to stop frying. Nothing is worse that having to clean grease out of dishes and off of walls.

Okay, so my pep talk above is not convincing. You and I love the taste of fried foods and don't want to give them up. There are several ways to enjoy a reasonable facsimile of fried foods without the fat or the mess. I am a really lazy cook so I prefer oven-frying. It is not messy at all and you don't have to watch the food constantly. A baking sheet (lined with foil if you want to really cut down on clean up) is coated with no-stick cooking spray. The food is added in a single layer and is given a light coating of cooking spray as well. It is then baked at 400-425 degrees. The food needs to be turned half way through the cooking time, which will vary depending on the size and type of food. Vegetables, chicken and fish can be breaded before oven-frying. Dip them briefly into ¼ cup water mixed with ¼ cup fat-free egg substitute, then into crumbs. Dry seasoned bread crumbs, corn flake crumbs and crushed dry stuffing crumbs all make good coatings. If you want just a bit of oil, add from 1 teaspoon to 1 tablespoon of vegetable oil to the egg mixture. When divided by several portions it will only add a few fat grams to each serving.

Sautéing and stir-frying are also forms of frying that are particularly great for cooking healthy. The foods are quickly cooked in a skillet or wok coated with no-stick cooking spray. Stir-fried foods are usually cut into small pieces of uniform size so they cook in minutes. Both sautéing and stir-frying are excellent ways to keep delicious taste and texture in food without added fat. However, don't think that the stir-fried dishes and sautéed dishes available in restaurants are low in fat. Many of them are cooked in lots of oil. When eating out ask that your sautéed and stir-fried entrees be prepared with very little or no fat added.

Quick-Cooking Vegetables And Grains By Steaming Or Microwaving

While the time-honored way of cooking vegetables in boiling water is okay, it is not the most nutritious nor the quickest method. Vital nutrients can be lost in the cooking water and vegetables can come out soggy and limp if boiled too long. In addition to sautéing and stir-frying, steaming and microwaving are terrific ways to cook vegetables. Since they are not submersed in water, the nutrients remain in the food, which also retains texture and taste. Steaming and microwaving are also exceptionally quick, which is a terrific bonus.

Food can be easily steamed with a deep, covered pot and an inexpensive steam rack. However, electric steamers that are controlled by a timer are very affordable. Because they turn themselves off, they do not have to be watched. This is a real plus since you can leave the kitchen without having to worry about overcooking the food. You can select a basic electric steamer or one that has various compartments for steaming more than one food at a time.

Although most homes now have microwave ovens, statistics indicate that they are mainly used to reheat meals or to make popcorn. If you don't use your microwave to cook vegetables, you should really try it. Microwaving is probably the simplest and best way to cook many vegetables. They don't have to be watched, they can't overcook if you time them correctly and they retain their nutrients. Of course, they also taste wonderful when correctly cooked in the microwave.

To steam or microwave vegetables, the pieces should be of fairly uniform size. If you plan to steam your food on the stove-top, select a deep pot with a lid. Add several inches of water, put the food in a steamer basket and place the basket in the pot. Make sure the water does not touch the food. Cover the pot and place over medium heat. Start counting the cooking time when wisps of steam can be seen rising from the pot. Do not let all of the water boil away. Add more if needed.

Microwaving is even more simple. Place the food in a covered microwave-proof dish along with several tablespoons of water and set the timer. Both the microwave and the electric steamer do practically everything but wash the dish for you.

If you cook vegetables the old-fashioned way in boiling water, ham or chicken bouillon cubes are great seasonings to add to the water during cooking. However, if you microwave or steam, the food is not submersed in the water. Therefore, they are best seasoned after cooking with a little granulated bouillon powder, fat-free margarine or a sauce. If you use fat-free margarine, the liquid kind works especially well. You may also wish to add additional seasoning along with the margarine. Garlic or other herbs, powdered crab spices and lemon juice are also flavorful additions.

Vegetable Steaming And Microwaving Chart

Times shown are for trimmed and cut up vegetables cooked tender-crisp. Time may vary depending on the wattage of your microwave or on whether you use an electric or stovetop steamer.

Vegetable	Amount	Steamed	Microwaved
Artichokes	1 pound	30 minutes	6-7 minutes
Asparagus	1 pound	8 minutes	6-7 minutes
Beets	1 pound	30 minutes	8 minutes
Broccoli	1 pound	10-15 minutes	8 minutes
Brussels Sprouts	1 pound	15 minutes	8 minutes
Cabbage	1 head	15 minutes	10 minutes
Carrots	1 pound	15 minutes	10 minutes
Cauliflower	1 head	10 minutes	10 minutes
Corn	4 ears	8-10 minutes	7 minutes
Eggplant	1 pound	10 minutes	7 minutes
Green Beans	1 pound	12 minutes	10 minutes
Green Peas	1 pound	10 minutes	7 minutes
Green Peppers	1 pound	10 minutes	6 minutes
Onions	1 pound	15 minutes	7 minutes
Potatoes	2 potatoes	30 minutes	7 minutes

Section Three:
The Recipes

Come Feast Along With Me

Now we get to the meat and potatoes of low-fat living—the recipes. Okay, so that's another bad pun, but those of you who aren't familiar with low-fat eating may really be under the impression that meat and potatoes are bad for you, especially if you are trying to lose weight. They aren't bad for you at all. You just have to learn how to prepare them properly. If you look at the following recipes and the recipes in *Live! Don't Diet!,* you will see that they are for real food. There is no pureed broccoli or boiled codfish. I couldn't eat that way for the rest of my life and neither can you.

These are more of the recipes that my husband Ken and I enjoyed while losing a total of 270 pounds. They not only helped us lose it, they help us keep it off because they are the recipes we live with day in and day out. There is good reason that we find them so easy to live with. Unlike dieting, which requires major deprivation, much lengthy preparation and the purchase of special ingredients, living a low-fat lifestyle allows us to eat like normal people, only healthier. We can have pizza or cheesecake or our favorite gooey casseroles. It is wonderful to be able to eat this way and still lose weight and maintain our good health.

In addition, you will be amazed at how much easier you will find preparing low-fat meals. If you are like me, you don't have a lot of time to spend in the kitchen so you will particularly like the fact that these low-fat dishes are quick and easy. There are no exotic, hard to find ingredients to buy and many of the dishes can be prepared in a very short time.

I have deliberately not used brand names in my ingredients list because brand names vary widely throughout the country. Even major food producers sell the same products under different labels in different areas. Nothing is more frustrating than looking for a brand called for in a recipe only to find that it is not available. The important thing is to read the label and make sure the brand you use is fat-free or low in fat.

I like to think of my recipes as road maps. In other words, they will get you where you are going. Prepared according to directions, they will result in tasty, filling, low-fat dishes. However, some of you may like to take little detours off the beaten path, so change the recipes to suit yourself. Feel free to do whatever you want, as long as any ingredient you add is low in fat. After all, they are just recipes, not something carved in stone.

I have listed only the fat grams with each recipe. I personally don't like to see the calorie content. That reminds me too much of a diet. Since I don't count calories, they are not of great concern to me if the recipe is a healthy, low-fat one. However, some people want to know the calorie content of their meals. For those who want this information, I have listed it at the end of the recipe section.

These are not just my recipes, now they are your recipes. You can impress your family and friends with just how tasty eating healthy can be—and just think of the thanks you'll get when you tell them you are cooking low-fat because you care about them and their good health. So you have friends or family who would rather fall dead than eat something healthy? Well, don't tell them that what they are eating is low in fat. They'll probably never know the difference and you will know you are helping them. So, come feast along with me!

Breakfast Recipes

Breakfast Sweet Roll Taste-Alikes

I have a real weakness for pastries. I am often tempted to leap the bakery counter, grab a few dozen goodies and stuff them into my mouth. However, I control myself because I know I can make something at home to satisfy my craving. While some of the pastries sold commercially may be relatively low in fat, they are still often loaded with sugar and calories. Since I can seldom eat just one, I prefer make my own reduced-calorie version at home.

The fat-free cinnamon roll recipe in *Live! Don't Diet!* has seen me through many tough times, especially after shopping. Grocery stores all seem to have full service bakeries these days. The wonderful smell of freshly baked sweet rolls and other goodies permeates the air. This usually sends me into a frenzy that can only be satisfied by a sweet treat.

If I don't have time or inclination to make my healthier homemade version, I'll make what I call a taste-alike. Maybe it doesn't taste exactly the same as the real thing, but it's close enough. You can do the same at breakfast or at any time you crave a pastry. Just think for a moment—what is a pastry? It is usually a form of yeast roll topped by a gooey, sweet filling and a sugary glaze. You can get much the same taste sensation by using plain old reduced-calorie bread. After all, the real sweet roll dough is just another variation of basic yeast and flour—in other words, bread. Okay, so we're not talking haute cuisine here but it does the trick. It will help satisfy that craving for the pastry you think you can't live without. Try some of these toppings for pastry taste-alikes:

- To make a fruit pastry taste-alike, spread a slice of reduced-calorie bread with your favorite reduced-sugar preserves. To make the glaze, blend several packets of aspartame-based sugar substitute with a few drops of water or fruit juice and drizzle over the top. For real overkill, squirt on some fat-free whipped topping.

- To make a cheese Danish taste-alike, spread a slice of reduced-calorie bread with the Cheesy Breakfast Burrito filling (see index) and drizzle on sugar substitute glaze.

- To make a cinnamon roll taste-alike, lightly spray your bread with fat-free, butter-flavored spray or squirt on liquid fat-free margarine. Sprinkle on a few raisins, then granulated aspartame-based sugar substitute and cinnamon to taste. Top with the sugar substitute glaze.

- To make a real monster taste-alike pastry, spread the bread with the Cheesy Breakfast Burrito filling, add your favorite jam or preserves, top with the sugar substitute glaze and add a bit of fat-free whipped topping.

The possibilities for making sweet roll taste-alikes are as limitless as your imagination. Experiment to your heart's content. The next time you are driven to contemplate buying a dozen of every sweet roll in the bakery case at your grocery, smile smugly to yourself and pass on by. You know that you can have your very own version at home without the guilt.

Cheesy Breakfast Burrito

We are all familiar with the breakfast burritos served at our favorite fast food restaurants. They are easy to make at home. One advantage to eating a breakfast burrito is that they are portable if you are in a hurry. The filling can be made in quantity and kept in the refrigerator. These burritos could also serve as a dessert in the evening. The filling of a breakfast burrito can change to suit your mood or what you have on hand. Scrambled egg substitute with a bit of minced low-fat ham and fat-free shredded Cheddar cheese is also good.

For each burrito:
1 fat-free flour tortilla
2 tablespoons fat-free cream cheese, softened
1 tablespoon fat-free sour cream
3 packets granulated aspartame-based sugar substitute
2 teaspoons low-sugar jam or preserves

Combine the cream cheese, sour cream and sugar substitute. Heat the tortilla in the microwave oven for approximately 10 seconds to soften. Spread the filling down the center of the tortilla, leaving 1" without filling at the top and bottom. Spoon the jam over the filling. Fold the unfilled top and bottom of the tortilla over the filling and roll the tortilla up, so that the filling is completely enclosed. Heat for another 10 seconds in the microwave oven, if desired.

1 serving
0 fat grams per serving

Cottage Cheese Pancakes

It amazes me that cottage cheese can be the primary ingredient in pancakes. I like this recipe because the cottage cheese adds protein. Also, a half cup of fat-free cottage cheese only has 80 calories, while a half cup of flour has about 200 calories. As I often say, I don't count calories but if I can reduce the calories in a recipe, I will. In this recipe, the 1½ cups of cottage cheese has 240 calories, in contrast to 600 calories in the 1½ cups of flour that a recipe for regular pancakes might contain.

½ cup fat-free egg substitute
1½ cups fat-free cottage cheese
¼ cup all-purpose flour
1 teaspoon sugar
No-stick cooking spray

Combine the egg substitute and cottage cheese. Gradually add the flour and sugar. Bake on a griddle that has been coated with no-stick cooking spray.

Variation: Add grated orange peel, grated apple, blueberries or sliced banana to the uncooked pancakes just after the batter is poured on the griddle.

8 pancakes
0 grams of fat per serving

Ham And Cheese Breakfast Casserole

This is a dish that is equally good for breakfast, lunch or dinner. As an added bonus it can be prepared the day before and refrigerated so that the only thing left to do is put it in the oven an hour before mealtime. Fresh fruit is a good accompaniment for the morning meal, while a vegetable salad goes well if it is served at dinner. Be sure to read the labels on the packaged croutons at your store. The brand I use has 8 fat grams per cup.

2 cups packaged garlic and cheese-flavored croutons
1 cup fat-free Cheddar cheese, shredded
4 ounces 98% fat-free ham, finely minced
1 medium onion, finely minced
2 cups skim milk
1 cup fat-free egg substitute
Light salt and pepper to taste

Combine the croutons, cheese, ham and onion. Place in a 8" x 8" baking dish that has been coated with no-stick cooking spray. Mix the milk, egg substitute, salt and pepper together and pour over the crouton mixture in the baking dish. Bake at 325 degrees for 50 minutes or until a knife inserted into the center comes out clean.

4 servings
5 fat grams per serving

Pancake Taste-Alikes

Not only is it easy to prepare homemade fat-free pancakes, many commercially prepared varieties in the frozen food section of the grocery are quite low in fat. However, sometimes we don't have time to make homemade pancakes and there are none in the freezer. This usually occurs at my house about the time all the pancake mix manufacturers choose to run advertisements on television featuring an actor attacking mounds of pancakes dripping with syrup and butter. When this happens, it makes me wish I could reach right into the TV and grab those pancakes right off the actor's plate. Instead, I'll just fool my mouth by making a stack of pancake taste-alikes.

Remember what I told you about sweet rolls? Right! They are just a variation on the same yeast and flour mixture that bread is made from. The same is essentially true of pancakes. The main ingredients are flour and a leavening agent, just like bread. Therefore, I just whip out my trusty loaf of reduced-calorie bread and make believe the slices are pancakes. Believe me, it works! My brain may know they aren't real pancakes, but my taste buds are satisfied. Here are a few pancake taste-alikes I rely on:

- Warm several slices of reduced-calorie bread for a few seconds in the microwave. Pour on liquid fat-free margarine and sugar-free syrup.

- For banana pancake taste-alikes, thinly slice ½ of a medium banana and mound it on reduced-calorie bread slices. Sprinkle the banana with a little cinnamon and granulated sugar substitute, pop it into the microwave briefly to warm it, then top with the liquid fat-free margarine and sugar-free syrup. This also works well using cooked apple slices instead of banana.

Sometimes I yearn for more elaborate pancakes. Remember all of those forbidden treats that pancake houses serve? Pancakes topped with sugar, fresh strawberries and whipped cream. Pancakes rolled around link sausages. I could go on forever since they have a million variations on the good old pancake—all loaded with fat and sugar. Everyone has their own personal favorites.

With a little creativity, it is easy to make our own low-fat version of almost any pancake house specialty, using our homemade pancakes, frozen pancakes or our pancake taste-alike, bread.

Potato-Crusted Breakfast Pie

If your family is accustomed to weekday breakfasts of cold cereal, they will be delighted if you serve this as a special weekend breakfast.

The crust:
2 large, potatoes, peeled and shredded
1 tablespoon all-purpose flour
¼ cup fat-free egg substitute
Light salt and pepper to taste
No-stick cooking spray

The filling:
1 cup fat-free Cheddar cheese, shredded
2 cups fat-free cottage cheese
4 ounces 98% fat-free ham, cubed
½ cup fat-free egg substitute
Light salt and pepper to taste

Prepare the crust by combining the potatoes, flour, egg substitute, salt and pepper. Press into a pie pan that has been coated with no-stick cooking spray. Bake, unfilled, for 15 minutes at 400 degrees. While the potato crust is baking, combine all of the filling ingredients. Remove the crust from the oven and top with the filling. Lower the oven temperature to 350 degrees and bake an additional 30 minutes.

4 servings
2 fat grams per serving

Appetizers

Baked Bean Dip

Surprisingly, most brands of baked beans are low in fat, despite the pork cooked with them. Just be sure to discard the pork and also check the label to make sure the brand you use is low in fat.

2 15-ounce cans fat-free vegetarian-style baked beans
1 medium onion, finely minced
1 green bell pepper, finely minced
2 teaspoons imitation bacon bits

Puree the baked beans in a blender or food processor. Add the remaining ingredients. May be served warm or at room temperature.

8 servings
1 fat gram per serving

Chunky Bean Spread

A popular restaurant near my home serves a similar spread to diners as they await their meal.

1 15-ounce can red beans, rinsed and drained
3 tablespoons sweet pickle relish
½ medium onion, finely minced
3 tablespoons fat-free mayonnaise
3 tablespoons fat-free sour cream

Combine all of the ingredients. Serve chilled as a spread with fat-free crackers, melba toast, or rye-crisp or serve on a bed of lettuce as a salad.

4 servings
0 fat grams per serving

Creamy Salsa Spread

This is good spread on crackers or as a dip with fat-free potato chips, pretzels or raw vegetables.

1 cup fat-free mayonnaise
1 cup fat-free sour cream
1 12-ounce jar mild or medium chunky salsa
½ medium onion, finely minced

Combine all ingredients. Serve chilled.

24 servings
0 fat grams per serving

Don't Give Up The Chip

A variation on the cinnamon and sugar sprinkled chips that many Mexican fast food restaurants offer as dessert.

10 fat-free flour tortillas
Butter-flavored no-stick cooking spray
Cinnamon to taste
Granulated aspartame-based sugar substitute to taste
Honey or sugar-free maple-flavored syrup

Cut each tortilla into 8 wedges. Place them in a single layer on a baking sheet that has been coated with no-stick cooking spray. Lightly spray the tops of the wedges with no-stick cooking spray. Sprinkle each one with cinnamon and sugar substitute to taste. Bake at 400 degrees for about 5 minutes or until the chips are lightly browned and crisp. Serve with honey or sugar-free maple-flavored syrup.

10 servings
0 fat grams per serving

Heavenly Fruit And Cheese Spread

Dried fruit and cheese make an interesting and appealing combination.

1 cup fat-free Cheddar cheese, shredded
½ cup dried apricots, finely chopped
½ cup pitted dates, chopped
½ cup golden raisins
½ cup boiling water
1 8-ounce package fat-free cream cheese, softened
⅓ cup skim milk

Allow the Cheddar cheese to come to room temperature. Combine the apricots, dates and raisins. Pour the boiling water over them and set aside. In a separate bowl, combine the cream cheese, the Cheddar cheese and milk. Drain the fruit and add it to the cheese mixture. Serve with fat-free wheat crackers.

8 servings
0 fat grams per serving

Herbed Cream Cheese Spread

2 8-ounce packages fat-free cream cheese, softened
2 teaspoons garlic powder or 2 cloves garlic, minced
½ teaspoon dried oregano
¼ teaspoon dried dillweed
¼ teaspoon dried basil
2 tablespoons dehydrated minced onion flakes

Combine the cream cheese, garlic, oregano, dillweed, basil and onion flakes. Serve chilled.

8 servings
0 fat grams per serving

Snappy Crackers

These crackers are not only a tasty snack, but are also terrific served as a topping for soup or salad.

No-stick butter-flavored cooking spray
1 16-ounce package oyster crackers, fat-free if available
1 envelope dry Ranch salad dressing mix

Coat a baking sheet with low sides with cooking spray. Place a layer of crackers on the baking sheet. Lightly coat the crackers with the cooking spray. Stir the crackers and lightly spray again. Sprinkle the crackers with the salad dressing mix and stir to coat. Bake the crackers for 45 minutes at 275 degrees, or until they are lightly browned. Store in an airtight container.

36 crackers per serving
0 fat grams per serving

Tangy Shrimp Spread

2 8-ounce packages fat-free cream cheese, softened
1 7-ounce can shrimp, rinsed and drained
½ medium onion, finely minced
No-stick cooking spray
½ cup bottled cocktail sauce

Combine the softened cream cheese, shrimp and onion. Pack into a small mold or bowl that has been coated with no-stick cooking spray. Chill until firm. Unmold on a serving plate that has been lined with lettuce. Spoon the cocktail sauce over the shrimp mold. Serve with fat-free crackers.

8 servings
1 fat gram per serving

Soups

Almost Effortless Ravioli Stew

Surprisingly, one of the most popular brands of commercially prepared canned cheese ravioli is now fat-free. This hearty stew, made with canned ravioli, is popular with children and adults as well. It can be made in minutes, which is a definite bonus.

1 medium onion, chopped
1 bell pepper, chopped
No-stick cooking spray
2 15-ounce cans Italian-style tomato sauce
1 15-ounce can sliced mushrooms, drained
2 15-ounce cans fat-free cheese ravioli
Fat-free Parmesan cheese

Sauté the onion and bell pepper in a skillet that has been coated with no-stick cooking spray. Place the onions, green pepper, tomato sauce and mushrooms in a large saucepan. Add the ravioli. Simmer for 15 minutes. Top individual portions with Parmesan cheese.

8 servings
0 fat grams per serving

Chunky Potato Soup

This is a recipe that can easily be changed to suit your taste. Use chopped broccoli instead of spinach if you like. A little 98% fat-free chopped ham or some sliced fat-free wieners can also be added.

1 large onion, chopped
2 stalks celery, chopped
No-stick cooking spray
2 15-ounce cans low-sodium, fat-free chicken broth
4 medium potatoes, peeled and chopped
1 10-ounce package frozen chopped spinach
2 cups skim milk
⅓ cup all-purpose flour
Light salt and pepper to taste (optional)

Sauté the onion and celery until tender in a large saucepan that has been coated with no-stick cooking spray. Add the chicken broth, potatoes and spinach. Bring to a boil, then lower the heat and simmer for 30 minutes or until the potatoes are tender. In a mixing bowl, gradually add the flour to the skim milk and stir until the flour is dissolved. Gradually add the milk to the simmering soup, stirring constantly. Simmer for 10 more minutes or until slightly thickened. Add light salt and pepper, if desired.

8 servings
0 fat grams per serving

Hearty White Chili

Serve topped with fat-free sour cream and chopped onion. Complete the white color scheme if you like by adding a little fat-free shredded mozzarella cheese as a topping. On the other hand, if you would like to add a little color, sprinkle on fat-free shredded Cheddar cheese and some chopped green onion, including the green tops. Cornbread is a hearty and delicious bread to offer on the side.

1 medium onion, finely chopped
3 15-ounce cans Great Northern beans
2 cups cooked boneless, skinless chicken breast, diced
1 15-ounce can low-sodium chicken broth
1 small can chopped chili peppers, mild or medium
2 teaspoons garlic powder
2 teaspoons cumin
Light salt and pepper to taste (optional)

Toppings:
Fat-free sour cream
Chopped onion or green onion, including green tops
Fat-free shredded mozzarella or Cheddar cheese

In a saucepan, combine the onions, beans, chicken, chicken broth, chili peppers, garlic powder, cumin, light salt and pepper to taste (optional). Simmer for 15 minutes. Ladle into individual soup bowls and add toppings.

4 servings
2 fat grams per serving

Smoky Pea Soup

I never really paid much attention to the packages of dried split peas I saw in the dried bean section at my local grocery store until my Mom served me a bowl of delicious split pea soup one chilly day. Now it's a favorite at my house, especially when served with hot cornbread.

8 cups water
2 cups dried split peas, soaked overnight and drained
1 15-ounce can low-sodium chicken broth
6 carrots, thinly sliced
1 medium onion, chopped
3 stalks celery, chopped
5 fat-free wieners, sliced
½ teaspoon liquid smoke
Light salt and pepper to taste (optional)

In a large saucepan, combine the water, split peas and chicken broth. Bring to a boil, lower the heat and simmer, covered, for 1 hour. Add the carrots, onion, celery, wieners, light salt and pepper. Simmer 30 additional minutes.

8 servings
1 fat gram per serving

Terrific Taco Soup

One evening when I was serving a thick, chili-flavored bean soup for dinner, I had some shredded lettuce on hand that I needed to use. Instead of making salad, I topped the soup with the lettuce and other Mexican-style taco toppings. It tasted somewhat like tacos, but was much easier to eat!

3 15-ounce cans chili beans
2 15-ounce cans Mexican-style chunky tomato sauce
1 medium onion, chopped
1 bell pepper, chopped
6 ounces browned ground round, rinsed and patted dry
6 fat-free corn tortillas
No-stick cooking spray
½ head iceberg lettuce, finely shredded
1 cup fat-free sour cream
1 mild onion, finely chopped
1 cup fat-free Cheddar cheese, shredded
1 cup mild or medium salsa

Combine the chili beans, tomato sauce, onion, bell pepper and ground round. Simmer for 30 minutes, or until the onion and the bell pepper are tender. Meanwhile cut each tortilla into 8 wedges and place on a baking sheet that has been coated with no-stick cooking spray. Bake at 350 degrees for 15 minutes, or until crisp. Ladle the soup into individual soup bowls. Top each portion with shredded lettuce, sour cream, chopped onion, shredded cheese and salsa. Serve with the tortilla wedges.

6 servings
4 fat grams per serving

Vegetable Soup With A Kick

Some people prefer meatless vegetable soup, while others like meat in it. This recipe is flexible. I use chicken, but 6 ounces of browned ground round that has been rinsed and patted dry is also good. It is equally delicious without any meat. Don't forget the cornbread! It is a must when you are serving vegetable soup.

2 cups cooked boneless, skinless chicken breast meat, diced
2 large onions, chopped
2 large potatoes, peeled and cubed
4 carrots, thinly sliced
1 48-ounce can vegetable juice
1 15-ounce can tomatoes with chili peppers, undrained
2 10-ounce packages frozen baby lima beans, thawed
2 15-ounce cans whole kernel corn, drained
Louisiana hot sauce to taste (optional)
Chopped raw onion (optional)

Combine the chicken, onions, potatoes, carrots, vegetable juice, tomatoes, lima beans and corn in a slow cooker. Cook for 10-12 hours on low. Top individual portions with Louisiana hot sauce to taste and chopped raw onion, if desired.

12 servings
2 fat grams per serving

Warm, Cozy Cream Of Tomato Soup

This is a comfort food from my childhood. My mother still makes it regularly for me—only now she makes a fat-free version.

2 medium onions, finely chopped
No-stick cooking spray
6 tablespoons all-purpose flour
4 cups skim milk
2 15-ounce cans tomatoes, chopped
Light salt and pepper to taste (optional)

In a large saucepan coated with no-stick cooking spray, sauté the onion. When tender, add the flour. Gradually stir in the milk. When the mixture is slightly thickened, add the tomatoes and their juice. Add light salt and pepper to taste (optional).

4 servings
0 fat grams per serving

Salads

Baked Bean Salad

1 head iceberg lettuce, shredded
2 16-ounce cans vegetarian-style baked beans, drained
1 mild onion, chopped
4 ounces 98% fat-free ham, chopped
1 cup fat-free Cheddar cheese, shredded
Fat-free Thousand Island or Ranch salad dressing

Arrange a bed of shredded lettuce on 4 dinner plates. Meanwhile, heat the baked beans until warmed through. Top the lettuce with beans, followed by salad dressing to taste. Add chopped onion, chopped ham and shredded Cheddar cheese.

4 servings
1 fat gram per serving

Cheesy Italian Potato Salad

4 large potatoes, peeled, cubed and boiled
1 medium onion, finely chopped
2 stalks celery, finely chopped
1 cup fat-free cottage cheese
½ cup fat-free sour cream
1 teaspoon garlic powder
1 teaspoon dried oregano
Light salt and pepper to taste (optional)
1 cup fat-free mozzarella cheese

Combine all of the ingredients. Gently toss to coat the vegetables. Serve chilled.

8 servings
0 fat grams per serving

Cool Summer Salad

1 head green cabbage, finely shredded
8 ounces 98% fat-free ham, chopped
1 medium onion, chopped
2 carrots, shredded
1 cup fat-free Swiss or mozzarella cheese
1 ounce bleu cheese, crumbled
1 cup fat-free mayonnaise
Light salt and pepper to taste (optional)

Combine the cabbage, ham, onion, carrots and Swiss or mozzarella cheese. In a mixing bowl, combine the bleu cheese and mayonnaise. Add to the cabbage mixture and toss to combine. Add light salt and pepper to taste (optional). Chill for at least 15 minutes to combine the flavors.

4 servings
3 fat grams per serving

Creamy Strawberry Salad

1 15-ounce can juice-packed crushed pineapple
1 large (8-serving) size fat-free, sugar-free strawberry gelatin
2 cups low-fat buttermilk
1 8-ounce carton fat-free whipped topping

Place the pineapple and juice in a saucepan and bring to a boil over medium heat. Add the gelatin and stir until it is completely dissolved. Let the dissolved gelatin cool to room temperature. When cool, add the buttermilk. Place the mixture in the refrigerator and chill until slightly thickened. Add the whipped topping and fold in gently. Chill until firm.

10 servings
0 fat grams per serving

Crisp Apple Slaw

1 head green cabbage, finely chopped or shredded
4 unpeeled red apples, cored and coarsely chopped
4 tablespoons dark raisins
1 cup fat-free mayonnaise
6 packets aspartame-based sugar substitute
⅓ cup lemon juice

Combine the cabbage, apples and raisins. In a separate mixing bowl, combine the mayonnaise, sugar substitute and lemon juice. Add the dressing to the cabbage mixture and toss to coat. Serve chilled.

10 servings
0 fat grams per serving

Crunchy Apple Salad

This salad is delicious served with ham or turkey.

3 large red apples, cored and cut into bite-size pieces
3 large green apples, cored and cut into bite-size pieces
3 large stalks celery, coarsely chopped
¼ cup raisins
½ cup fat-free mayonnaise
3 packets aspartame-based sugar substitute
2 tablespoons lemon juice

Combine the apples, celery and raisins in a serving bowl. In a separate bowl, combine the mayonnaise, sugar substitute and lemon juice. Add the mayonnaise mixture to the apple mixture and toss gently. Serve chilled.

8 servings
0 fat grams per serving

Delicious Layered Slaw

Layered salads, prepared in advance, frosted with a mayonnaise-based dressing, and tossed at serving time have been popular for quite a while. It is easy to see why. They are easy to prepare, pretty and very tasty. The concept works equally well with cole slaw.

1 head green cabbage, shredded
3 medium potatoes, peeled, cubed and boiled
1 10-ounce package frozen English peas, thawed, rinsed and
    drained
1 medium onion, chopped
4 hard-boiled eggs, whites only, chopped
1 bell pepper, chopped
1 cup fat-free mayonnaise
2 tablespoons cider vinegar
2 packets sugar substitute

In a clear glass serving dish, place a layer of cabbage, a layer of potatoes, a layer of peas, a layer of chopped onion, a layer of egg whites and a layer of green pepper. Repeat the layers. In a mixing bowl, combine the mayonnaise, vinegar and sugar substitute. Spread the mixture over the slaw. Cover and refrigerate until serving time. Before serving, toss the ingredients to combine.

8 servings
0 fat grams per serving

Delightful Frozen Fruit Salad

1 8-ounce package fat-free cream cheese, softened
½ cup skim milk
4 packets aspartame-based sugar substitute
1 15-ounce can juice-packed fruit cocktail, undrained

Combine the cream cheese, skim milk and sugar substitute. Add the fruit cocktail. Place the mixture in a serving dish and freeze until firm. Allow to stand at room temperature for about 10 minutes before serving,

4 servings
0 fat grams per serving

Holiday Cranberry Salad

1 large (8-serving size) box sugar-free strawberry gelatin
1 ½ cups boiling water
1 8-ounce can juice-packed crushed pineapple, drained, juice
　 reserved
½ cup unsweetened orange juice
2 cups fresh cranberries
1 medium apple, peeled, cored and sliced

Place the gelatin in a large mixing bowl. Add the boiling water and stir until dissolved. Add the reserved pineapple juice and the orange juice. Chill until it is slightly thickened. Meanwhile, chop the cranberries and apple in a blender or food processor. Add the fruits to the gelatin mixture and place in a serving dish or mold. Chill until firm.

8 servings
0 fat grams per serving

Jellied Fresh Fruit Salad

This is a very refreshing and pretty salad. For maximum effect, serve unmolded on a bed of leaf lettuce or in a clear class serving dish.

1 large (8-serving size) box fat-free, sugar-free orange gelatin
3 cups water, divided
1 8-ounce can juice-packed pineapple tidbits, juice reserved
1 grapefruit, peeled, seeded and sectioned
2 oranges, peeled, seeded and sectioned
2 ripe bananas, thinly sliced
1 cup fresh strawberries, sliced

Place the gelatin in a large mixing bowl. In a saucepan, bring 2 cups of water to a boil. Add the boiling water to the gelatin and stir until the gelatin is completely dissolved. Combine the remaining 1 cup water and the reserved pineapple juice. Add to the gelatin. Refrigerate until the mixture is slightly thickened. Chop the grapefruit and orange sections into bite-size pieces. Add the pineapple, grapefruit, oranges, bananas and pineapple. Pour the mixture into a serving dish or mold and chill until firm.

12 servings
0 fat grams per serving

Killer Salsa Salad

Well, maybe it's not a killer but it will bowl diners over with its delicious spicy taste. Top with a dollop of fat-free sour cream and a sprinkle of finely chopped green onion. Fat-free tortilla chips are terrific served along with this salad.

1 15-ounce can stewed tomatoes
2 tablespoons cider vinegar
½ cup finely minced onion
1 bell pepper, finely minced
½ cup celery, finely minced
1 small can mild, medium or hot chopped chili peppers, drained
1 teaspoon Louisiana hot sauce
1 small (4-serving size) box sugar-free lemon gelatin

In a saucepan, combine the stewed tomatoes, vinegar, onion, bell pepper, celery, chili peppers and hot sauce. Bring the mixture to a boil over medium heat. Add the gelatin and stir until it has dissolved. Pour into a mold or serving dish and refrigerate until firm.

6 servings
0 fat grams per serving

Kind Of Greek Salad

Cottage cheese is a pretty good substitute for the feta cheese normally found in Greek salads. If you can't do without the feta, go ahead and use it in moderation. One ounce contains only 6 fat grams.

1 head iceberg lettuce, shredded
1 mild onion, sliced into thin rings
1 cucumber, thinly sliced
1 tomato, cut into wedges
½ cup fat-free cottage cheese
Fat-free Italian salad dressing
4 tablespoons fat-free Parmesan cheese, grated
Coarsely ground black pepper

Place a bed of shredded lettuce on individual salad plates. Scatter onion rings, cucumber slices and tomato wedges over lettuce. Top with a tablespoon of cottage cheese, then with Italian salad dressing. Sprinkle a tablespoon of Parmesan cheese and a bit of coarsely ground black pepper over the salad.

4 servings
0 fat grams per serving

Mexican Spinach Salad

1 1-pound bag fresh spinach, washed, stems removed and torn
   into bite-size pieces
1 medium onion, thinly sliced
1 cup sliced fresh mushrooms
1 cup fat-free Cheddar cheese, shredded
½ cup fat-free vinaigrette salad dressing
1 teaspoon chili powder
½ teaspoon cumin

Combine the spinach, onion, mushrooms and cheese.
Combine the salad dressing, chili powder and cumin. Toss with
the spinach mixture. Serve chilled.

4 servings
0 fat grams per serving

Secret Tuna Salad

My Mom has a friend who gave her a great secret tip for
making terrific tuna or chicken salad. Add a potato!

1 large baking potato, peeled and boiled
2 7-ounce cans white chunk tuna, water-packed
2 stalks celery, finely chopped
3 tablespoons sweet pickle relish
3 tablespoons fat-free mayonnaise
1 tablespoons prepared mustard

Refrigerate the potato until it is cold, then grate into a
mixing bowl. Add the tuna, celery, pickle relish, mayonnaise and
mustard. Mix gently until thoroughly combined.

8 servings
1 fat gram per serving

Snappy Green Bean Salad

3 15-ounce cans cut green beans, drained
2 medium potatoes, peeled, cubed and boiled
1 medium onion, chopped
½ cup fat-free mayonnaise
½ cup fat-free Italian salad dressing
Light salt and pepper to taste (optional)

Combine the green beans, potatoes, and onion. In a separate bowl, combine the mayonnaise, Italian dressing and light salt and pepper to taste (optional). Combine the vegetables and the dressing. Serve chilled.

8 servings
0 fat grams per serving

Summer In A Bowl

½ medium watermelon, seeded and cubed
1 cantaloupe, seeded and cubed
1 15-ounce can juice-packed pineapple tidbits, juice reserved
2 cups seedless red or green grapes
1 pint strawberries, hulled and sliced
4 fresh peaches, peeled, seeded and sliced
1 12-ounce can apricot nectar
2 tablespoons almond extract
6 packets aspartame-based sugar substitute

In a large serving bowl, combine the fruit. In a separate bowl, combine the apricot nectar, almond extract and sugar substitute. Add the apricot mixture to the fruit and toss gently. Allow to chill for several hours in the refrigerator.

12 servings
0 fat grams per serving

Beef Main Dishes

Acapulco Rice

Combining ground beef with rice and lots of vegetables is a good way to make a little meat go a long way.

3 stalks celery, chopped
1 pound fresh mushrooms, sliced
No-stick cooking spray
4 cups cooked rice
1 15-ounce can diced tomatoes with chilies, undrained
1 1-ounce package dehydrated onion soup mix
6 ounces brown ground round, rinsed and patted dry
1 cup fat-free sour cream
1 cup fat-free Cheddar cheese, shredded

Sauté the celery and mushrooms in a skillet that has been coated with no-stick cooking spray. When the vegetables are tender, add the rice, tomatoes, onion soup mix and ground round. In a casserole dish that has been coated with no-stick cooking spray, place ½ of the rice mixture. Spread the sour cream over the rice, then add the cheese. Top with the remaining rice mixture. Bake for 30 minutes at 350 degrees.

4 servings
3 fat grams per serving

Baked Beef And Pasta Supreme

There are loads of different shaped pastas on the market. Most of them can be used interchangeably in this recipe. Children especially might like wheel-shaped pasta or shell-shaped pasta. Tri-colored pasta would also be fun to use for a change.

1 12-ounce package small pasta shells, cooked and drained
6 ounces browned ground round, rinsed and patted dry
1 cup fat-free cottage cheese
1 cup fat-free mozzarella
1 tablespoon Italian seasoning blend
Light salt and pepper to taste (optional)
No-stick cooking spray
1 28-ounce jar commercially prepared fat-free
    spaghetti sauce
1 15-ounce can sliced mushrooms, drained
1 1-ounce package dehydrated onion soup mix
1 tablespoon grated fat-free Parmesan cheese

Combine the pasta shells, ground round, cottage cheese, mozzarella and Italian seasoning blend. Add light salt and pepper if desired. Place the mixture in a casserole dish that has been coated with no-stick cooking spray. Combine the spaghetti sauce, mushrooms and onion soup mix. Pour over the pasta. Bake at 350 degrees for 30 minutes. Top with the grated Parmesan cheese just before serving.

4 servings
4 fat grams per serving

Barbecue Pie

The wonderful zesty taste of barbecue has a natural affinity for cornbread.

1 large onion coarsely chopped
1 large green bell pepper, coarsely chopped
No-stick cooking spray
6 ounces browned ground round, rinsed and patted dry
1 cup fat-free barbecue sauce
1 cup cornmeal mix
½ cup fat-free cottage cheese
1 cup fat-free Cheddar, shredded
¼ cup fat-free egg substitute
1 cup water

Sauté the onion and green bell pepper in a skillet that has been coated with no-stick cooking spray. When the vegetables are tender, add the ground round and the barbecue sauce. Place the mixture in a casserole dish that has also been coated with no-stick cooking spray. Combine the cornmeal mix, cottage cheese, Cheddar cheese, egg substitute and water. Pour this mixture over the beef mixture. Bake for 30 minutes at 350 degrees.

4 servings
5 fat grams per serving

Chili Mountain

Children love this dish not only because it is different, but also because it contains many childhood favorites—macaroni, chili and cheese. Adults love it for the same reason. It is also fun when you have guests for a casual dinner. You can set out the ingredients and let guests build their own mountain.

3 15-ounce cans chili-style beans
2 15-ounce cans chunky Mexican-style tomato sauce
6 ounces browned ground round, rinsed and drained
1 16-ounce package elbow macaroni, prepared
   according to package directions
Finely shredded iceberg lettuce
1 onion, finely minced
1 cup fat-free sour cream
½ cup commercially prepared bottled salsa, hot or mild
1 cup fat-free Cheddar cheese, shredded

Combine the chili beans, tomato sauce and ground round in a saucepan. Simmer for 10 minutes. Meanwhile place a portion of the macaroni on 4 dinner plates. Top with the chili, followed by shredded lettuce, minced onion, sour cream, salsa and cheese.

4 servings
4 fat grams per serving

Country-Style Butterbean Pie

If you prefer, other beans, such as Great Northern beans or kidney beans can be used in this recipe. You can even combine a variety of your favorites.

4 cups cooked large white butterbeans
1 medium onion, coarsely chopped
1 medium potato, peeled and chopped
6 ounces browned ground round, rinsed and patted dry
1 15-ounce can tomato sauce
No-stick cooking spray
1 cup cornmeal mix
¼ cup fat-free egg substitute
1 cup water
1 tablespoon fat-free sour cream

Combine the butterbeans, onion, potato, ground round and tomato sauce. Place this mixture in a baking dish that has been coated with no-stick cooking spray. Combine the cornmeal mix, egg substitute, water and sour cream. Pour this mixture over the butterbean mixture. Bake for 45 minutes at 350 degrees.

4 servings
3 fat grams per serving

Creamy Pasta Casserole

1 12-ounce package elbow macaroni, prepared according to
    package directions
½ cup fat-free egg substitute, divided
1 cup skim milk
Light salt and pepper to taste (optional)
No-stick cooking spray
1 cup fat-free cottage cheese
¼ cup fat-free Parmesan cheese
2 cups commercially prepared fat-free spaghetti sauce
6 ounces browned ground round, rinsed and patted dry
1 15-ounce can mushrooms, drained

In a mixing bowl, combine the macaroni, ¼ cup egg substitute and the skim milk. Add the light salt and pepper, if desired. Place the mixture in a baking dish that has been coated with no-stick cooking spray. Combine the cottage cheese, Parmesan cheese and the remaining ¼ cup egg substitute. Pour this mixture over the pasta layer. Combine the spaghetti sauce, ground round and mushrooms. Spoon gently over the cottage cheese layer. Bake for 30 minutes at 350 degrees.

4 servings
3 fat grams per serving

Crunchy Potato-Beef Casserole

This recipe will be a hit with the meat and potatoes fans in the family.

2 large onions, chopped
1 large green pepper, chopped
No-stick cooking spray
6 ounces browned ground round, rinsed and patted dry
1 15-ounce can tomato sauce
1 1-ounce package dehydrated onion soup mix
1 package refrigerated or frozen shredded potatoes

Sauté the onion and green pepper in a skillet that has been coated with no-stick cooking spray. When the vegetables are tender, add the ground round, the tomato sauce and the onion soup mix. Place the mixture in a baking dish that has been coated with no-stick cooking spray. Top the meat mixture with the shredded potatoes. Lightly spray the potatoes with no-stick cooking spray. Bake for 30 minutes at 425 degrees.

4 servings
4 fat grams per serving

Dinnertime Sloppy Joes

Sloppy Joes are very good and very popular sandwiches. This dish goes a step further and serves them open-faced as an entree. Good with mashed potatoes and cole slaw on the side.

1 medium onion, chopped
No-stick cooking spray.
6 ounces browned ground round, rinsed and patted dry
1 10 ¾-ounce can low-fat beef gravy
1 15-ounce can mushrooms, drained
1 tablespoon ketchup
2 tablespoons fat-free sour cream
1 teaspoon garlic powder
4 reduced-calorie hamburger buns, split and toasted

Sauté the onion in a skillet that has been coated with no-stick cooking spray. When it is tender, add the ground round, beef gravy, mushrooms, ketchup, sour cream and garlic powder. Simmer until warmed through. Place two hamburger bun halves on each dinner plate. Top each half with the hamburger mixture.

4 servings
2 fat grams per serving

Extra-Easy Baked Eye Of Round Roast

1 2-pound eye of round roast, all visible fat removed
1 10¾-ounce can 97% fat-free cream of mushroom soup
½ cup water
1 1-ounce package dehydrated onion soup mix
1 teaspoon garlic powder

      Place a large piece of aluminum foil in a medium-sized baking dish. Place the roast in the center of the foil. Pull the sides of the foil up so that they surround the roast. Combine the mushroom soup, water, garlic powder and onion soup mix. Pour over the roast. Pull the aluminum foil up over the top and ends of the roast and fold so that the gravy cannot leak out. Bake the roast for 2 hours at 350 degrees. It will be well done.

8 servings, 6 fat grams per serving

Gourmet Steak

1 pound eye of round roast, all visible fat removed
1 teaspoon garlic powder
1 teaspoon Worcestershire sauce
No-stick cooking spray
6 green onions, including tops, chopped
1 15-ounce can sliced mushrooms, drained
1 10½-ounce can low-fat beef gravy

      Cut the eye of round into 4 4-ounce steaks. Sprinkle each steak with garlic powder and Worcestershire sauce. Sauté the beef in a skillet that has been coated with no-stick cooking spray until done to your preference. Meanwhile, combine the green onions, mushrooms and beef gravy in a small saucepan and simmer for 5 minutes. Place each steak on a dinner plate and top with several tablespoons of the gravy.

4 servings, 6 fat grams per serving

Onion Baked Steak

The flavors of onions and beef complement each other beautifully. The same can be said for onions and potatoes. This recipe can't help but please everyone since it combines all of these great tastes.

4 4-ounce top round steaks, trimmed of all visible fat
No-stick cooking spray
4 medium potatoes, peeled and cubed
1 10¾-ounce can condensed French onion soup
½ soup can water

Sauté the steaks in a skillet that has been coated with no-stick cooking spray for 5 minutes per side. When they are browned, remove them to a baking dish that has also been coated with no-stick cooking spray. Place the potatoes around the meat. Combine the onion soup and water. Pour the soup over the meat and potatoes. Cover and bake at 350 degrees for 45 minutes.

4 servings
5 fat grams per serving

Pizza Macaroni-Style

You and your family will like this unique twist on that old standby, pizza. Serve with a mixed green salad and Italian bread.

1 16-ounce package elbow macaroni, prepared according to
    package directions
No-stick cooking spray
1 cup skim milk
½ cup fat-free egg substitute
Light salt and pepper to taste
1 28-ounce can fat-free spaghetti sauce
6 ounces browned ground round, rinsed and patted dry
1 medium onion finely chopped
1 green pepper, finely chopped
1 cup fresh mushrooms, sliced
1 cup fat-free mozzarella cheese, shredded
4 tablespoons fat-free Parmesan cheese, grated

Spread the macaroni in a 9" x 13" baking dish that has been coated with no-stick cooking spray. Combine the milk, egg substitute, salt and pepper. Pour the mixture over the macaroni. Bake for 10 minutes at 350 degrees. Remove from the oven and spread the spaghetti sauce over the macaroni. Top with the ground round, onion and green pepper. Bake for 20 additional minutes. Remove from the oven and top with the mozzarella and Parmesan cheese. Serve immediately.

8 servings
3 fat grams per serving

Ken's Quick Stuffed Peppers

My husband Ken thought up this recipe one day when he found about a zillion bell peppers in our refrigerator. I think he wanted them out of the way, so he suggested I make low-fat stuffed peppers. They have been a regular meal on our menu ever since.

4 large bell peppers
1 box instant long grain and wild rice mix, made according
   to package directions, omitting margarine
6 ounces browned ground round, rinsed and drained
1 medium onion, chopped
1 15-ounce can tomato sauce
3 packets sugar substitute
1 tablespoon cider vinegar

Cut the bell peppers in half lengthwise, removing stems, pith and seeds. In a mixing bowl, combine the rice, ground round and onion. Spoon the rice mixture into the 8 pepper halves. Press the mixture down to tightly stuff the pepper. Place the pepper halves in a microwave-proof baking dish. Combine the tomato sauce, sugar substitute and vinegar. Pour over the stuffed peppers. Cover the baking dish loosely with plastic wrap. Microwave for 10 minutes on high. Let stand 5 minutes.

4 servings
4 fat grams per serving

Slow Cooker Oriental Beef

We usually equate oriental recipes with quick cooking since so many of them are stir-fried. This recipe is just the opposite. It cooks all day! It's even easier than stir-frying because it doesn't have to be watched.

1 pound top round, cut into cubes
1 large onion, chopped
1 6-ounce can tomato paste
½ cup water
1 8-ounce can juice packed pineapple tidbits, undrained
1 8-ounce can sliced water chestnuts, drained
¼ cup cider vinegar
3 packets sugar substitute
Hot, cooked rice

Place the meat, onion and water chestnuts in a slow cooker. In a mixing bowl, combine the tomato paste, water and undrained pineapple tidbits. Pour over the beef. Cook for 8-10 hours on low. Shortly before serving, add the vinegar and sugar substitute. Serve over rice.

4 servings
4 fat grams per serving

Spaghetti With A Difference

We usually think of serving spaghetti with a tomato-based sauce. However beef gravy makes a different and very good spaghetti sauce.

2 medium onions, coarsely chopped
No-stick cooking spray
2 10 ½-ounce cans low-fat beef gravy
1 15-ounce can sliced mushrooms, drained
6 ounces browned ground round, rinsed and patted dry
1 teaspoon garlic powder
1 16-ounce package angel hair pasta, prepared according to
   package directions

Sauté the onion in a skillet that has been coated with no-stick cooking spray. When the onion is tender, add the beef gravy, mushrooms, ground round and garlic powder. Simmer for 10 minutes. Meanwhile, place a portion on the cooked spaghetti on each dinner plate. Top the spaghetti with the heated sauce.

6 servings
4 fat grams per serving

Steak In A Stew

A cross between a steak dinner and beef stew which my family enjoys. This recipe can be simplified even more by using canned whole potatoes. They lose much of their canned taste in the cooking process.

4 4-ounce slices eye of round, all visible fat removed
No-stick cooking spray
4 medium baking potatoes, peeled and cubed
4 medium carrots, peeled and cut into 2" pieces
1 15-ounce can English peas, drained
1 15-ounce can sliced mushrooms, drained
1 10 ½-ounce can low-fat beef gravy
½ cup water
1 teaspoon garlic powder
Light salt and pepper to taste (optional)

Sauté the beef slices in a skillet that has been coated with no-stick cooking spray for 5 minutes per side. Remove to a baking dish that has also been coated with no-stick cooking spray. Arrange the vegetables around the meat. Combine the gravy, water, garlic powder, salt and pepper. Pour over the meat and vegetables. Cover and bake for 1 hour at 350 degrees.

4 servings
5 fat grams per serving

Steak Teriyaki

This teriyaki recipe has a different twist. It contains orange juice instead of pineapple juice. It can also be served with fruit, such as mandarin orange sections or pineapple tidbits, added to the sauce.

4 4-ounce cube steaks (top round)
No-stick cooking spray
1 cup unsweetened orange juice
2 tablespoons light soy sauce, low-sodium if desired
1 teaspoon garlic powder
1 tablespoon cornstarch
3 packets sugar substitute

Sauté the cube steaks in a skillet that has been coated with no-stick cooking spray. When cooked to your personal preference, remove to a platter. Combine the orange juice, soy sauce, garlic powder and cornstarch. Place the sauce ingredients in the skillet and cook over low heat until thickened, stirring frequently. Add the sugar substitute. Return the meat to the skillet and heat briefly.

4 servings
5 fat grams per serving

Tasty Tamale Pie

Cornmeal mixture:
4 cups water, divided
1 ½ cups cornmeal
1 tablespoon chili powder
1 teaspoon cumin
Light salt to taste

Filling:
6 ounces browned ground round, rinsed and patted dry
1 6-ounce can tomato paste
1 tablespoon each chili powder and cumin
1 cup water
1 medium onion, finely minced
1 15-ounce can whole kernel corn
No-stick cooking spray
1 15-ounce can chunky Mexican-style tomato sauce

Combine the cornmeal, chili powder, cumin and light salt. Slowly add 1 ½ cups cold water. Gradually add this mixture to the boiling water. Stir until thickened. For the filling, combine the ground round, tomato paste, spices, water, onion and corn. Pour half of the hot cornmeal mixture into an oblong baking dish that has been coated with no-stick cooking spray. When it has cooled slightly top with the filling ingredients. Pour the remaining cornmeal mixture over the filling. Cover and bake for 30 minutes at 350 degrees. Top portions with the heated tomato sauce.

12 servings
2 fat grams per serving

Chicken Main Dishes

Barbecued Chicken Casserole

Everyone in my family loves this because they are crazy about barbecue. I love it because it is a meal in one dish and cooks itself while I'm at work. Cole slaw makes a good accompaniment.

4 medium potatoes, peeled and cubed
2 medium onions, coarsely chopped
4 4-ounce chicken breast halves, boned and skinned, cut into
    bite-sized pieces
1 cup fat-free bottled barbecue sauce
1 1-ounce package dehydrated onion soup mix
½ cup water

Place the potatoes and onions in the bottom of a slow cooker. Place the chicken on top of the vegetables. Combine the barbecue sauce, onion soup mix and water. Pour over the vegetables and chicken. Cook on low for 8-10 hours. This may also be cooked in the oven, covered, for 1 hour at 350 degrees.

4 servings
4 fat grams per serving

Basic Lemon-Herb Broiled Chicken

1 tablespoon lemon juice
1 tablespoon vegetable oil
1 teaspoon garlic powder
1 teaspoon dried parsley flakes
1 teaspoon Worcestershire sauce
4 4-ounce chicken breast halves, skinned and boned
No-stick cooking spray
Light salt and pepper to taste (optional)

Combine the lemon juice, oil, garlic powder, parsley flakes and Worcestershire sauce. Place the chicken breasts in a baking dish that has been coated with no-stick cooking spray. Brush each breast with the basting sauce. Broil 7 minutes then turn and brush with the sauce. Broil an additional 7 minutes. Watch carefully. The exact cooking time will depend on the size and thickness of the chicken pieces.

4 servings
6 fat grams per serving

Chicken Italian

While real pepperoni has too much fat, 97% fat-free smoked sausage is close enough in taste to be an acceptable substitute, either on pizza or in this recipe.

No-stick cooking spray
4 4-ounce chicken breast halves, skinned and boned
1 onion, cut into wedges
½ pound 97% fat-free smoked sausage, thinly sliced
2 cups commercially prepared fat-free spaghetti sauce

Sauté the chicken breasts in a skillet that has been coated with no-stick cooking spray for 6 minutes on each side. Remove the chicken from the skillet. Sauté the onion and the smoked sausage until the sausage is lightly browned. Return the chicken to the skillet and add the spaghetti sauce. Simmer for 10 minutes.

4 servings
6 fat grams per serving

Chunky Chicken Hash

This is a not only a meal in one dish, it is a good way to use up some of the vegetables you have left in the refrigerator. Just add them to the basic recipe.

2 cups cooked chicken breast, cubed
4 medium potatoes, peeled, cubed and boiled
1 medium onion, coarsely chopped
1 10¾-ounce can 97% fat-free cream of mushroom soup
1 cup fat-free sour cream
Light salt and pepper to taste (optional)
No-stick cooking spray

Combine the chicken, potatoes, onion, mushroom soup, sour cream, light salt and pepper. Pour into a casserole dish that has been coated with no-stick cooking spray. Bake for 40 minutes, covered, at 350 degrees.

4 servings
5 fat grams per serving

Creamy Chicken Casserole

1 10-ounce package frozen chopped spinach, cooked and
   drained
¼ cup fat-free egg substitute
1 cup fat-free cottage cheese
½ cup fat-free Parmesan cheese
1 cup fat-free mozzarella cheese, shredded
1 12-ounce package medium noodles, prepared according to
   package directions
1 cup fat-free sour cream
Light salt and pepper to taste (optional)
1 cup cooked chicken breast, chopped
No-stick cooking spray

     Combine the spinach, egg substitute, cottage cheese, Parmesan cheese and mozzarella cheese. In a separate bowl, combine the cooked noodles, sour cream and chicken. Add light salt and pepper if desired. In a casserole dish that has been coated with no-stick cooking spray, place half of the noodles followed by half of the cheese mixture, then the remaining noodles, followed by the remaining cheese mixture. Bake, covered, for 30 minutes at 350 degrees.

4 servings
2 fat grams per serving

Crispy Oven Chicken

This is a different variation on that stand-by, oven-fried chicken. It is special enough to serve to company.

1 cup fat-free sour cream
1 tablespoon lemon juice
½ teaspoon garlic powder
Light salt and pepper to taste (optional)
6 4-ounce chicken breast halves, skinned and boned
2 cups packaged herb-seasoned stuffing crumbs
No-stick cooking spray

Combine the sour cream, lemon juice, and garlic powder. If desired add the light salt and pepper. Coat each chicken breast half with the mixture. After coating, roll each breast in the stuffing crumbs. If the crumbs are large, you may wish to crush them slightly before rolling the chicken in them. Place the chicken in a baking dish that has been coated with no-stick cooking spray. Lightly spray each breast with the cooking spray. Bake, uncovered, for 30 minutes at 400 degrees, until well browned. Do not overcook.

6 servings
5 fat grams per serving

Ham And Cheese Chicken

While the French call their classic dish Chicken Cordon Bleu, this variation, as well as the original, are basically combinations of those All-American favorites, ham, cheese and chicken.

4 4-ounce chicken breast halves, boned and skinned
No-stick cooking spray
Light salt and pepper to taste (optional)
4 extra-thin slices deli-style 98% fat-free ham
4 ¾-ounce slices fat-free Swiss or Cheddar cheese

Sauté the chicken in a skillet that has been coated with no-stick cooking spray for about 6 minutes each side. When the chicken is cooked, top with a slice of cheese and a slice of ham. Cover briefly to melt the cheese. Serve immediately.

4 servings
4 fat grams per serving

Helen's And Linda's Chicken Picante

My friend Helen Davis has lost 75 pounds since she began watching her fat intake. She got this super quick and easy recipe from her sister, Linda Mendel.

4 4-ounce boneless, skinless, chicken breast halves
    cut into bite-size pieces
No-stick cooking spray
1 20-ounce jar chunky picante sauce, mild or medium
Hot, cooked rice

Place the chicken in a baking dish that has been coated with no-stick cooking spray. Pour the picante sauce over the chicken. Bake, covered for 30 minutes at 350 degrees. Serve over hot, cooked rice.

4 servings
4 fat grams per serving

Mexican Grilled Chicken

1 teaspoon cider vinegar
¼ cup water
1 teaspoon ground chili powder
1 teaspoon ground cumin
1 teaspoon garlic powder
4 4-ounce chicken breasts, skinned and boned

Combine the vinegar, water, chili powder, cumin and garlic powder. Brush the chicken on both sides with the mixture. Grill for approximately 20 minutes.

4 servings
4 fat grams per serving

Pasta Jambalaya

A new way to enjoy the spicy flavors of the Louisiana classic, Jambalaya. Fresh shrimp can also be added, if desired, for an even more authentic version.

No-stick cooking spray
1 medium onion, coarsely chopped
1 bell pepper, coarsely chopped
3 stalks celery, coarsely chopped
1 cup cooked chicken breast, cubed
½ pound 97% fat-free smoked sausage, sliced
½ cup 98% fat-free ham, cubed
1 15-ounce can tomato sauce
1 tablespoon Cajun-style seasoning, commercially prepared or
    homemade (see recipe index)
1 12-ounce package angel hair pasta, prepared according
    to package directions

In a skillet that has been coated with no-stick cooking spray, sauté the onion, green pepper and celery until tender-crisp. Add the chicken, smoked sausage and ham and continue cooking for several minutes until the meats are slightly browned. Add the tomato sauce and the Cajun seasoning. Serve over angel hair pasta.

6 servings
5 fat grams per serving

Peachy Chicken Deluxe

I love the taste of fruit with chicken. Somehow their flavors seem to complement each other. Chinese Sweet and Sour Chicken is not the only way to enjoy the taste of chicken with fruit. This recipe is another.

No-stick cooking spray
6 4-ounce chicken breast halves, skinned and boned
1 onion, coarsely chopped
1 bell pepper, coarsely chopped
1 15-ounce can sliced peaches, packed in juice, juice reserved
¼ cup soy sauce
2 tablespoons lemon juice
1 tablespoon cornstarch
½ cup water

Sauté the chicken breasts in a skillet that has been coated with no-stick cooking spray for 6 minutes on each side. When they are cooked throughout and lightly brown, remove them from the skillet. In the same skillet, sauté the onion and peppers until they are tender-crisp. Remove the onion and peppers from the skillet. Drain the juice from the peaches into the skillet. Add the soy sauce and lemon juice. Combine the water and cornstarch and add to the skillet. Stir over low heat until the sauce has thickened. Add the sliced peaches to the sauce, as well as the reserved chicken and vegetables. Continue cooking for 5 minutes.

6 servings
4 fat grams per serving

Piquant Barbecued Chicken

We usually think of the traditional tomato-based sauce when we think of barbecue. However, this spicy sauce is just as good in its own way. Try it for a change.

1 tablespoon vegetable oil
2 tablespoons lemon juice
1 teaspoon dry mustard
1 tablespoon Worcestershire sauce
1 teaspoon garlic powder
¼ teaspoon Louisiana-style hot sauce
6 4-ounce chicken breasts, skinned and boned
No-stick cooking spray

Combine the oil, lemon juice, dry mustard, Worcestershire sauce, garlic powder and hot sauce. Place the chicken breasts on a grill that has been coated with no-stick cooking spray. Brush with the sauce. Grill for about 6 minutes per side, basting frequently with the sauce. Do not overcook.

6 servings
6 fat grams per serving

Quick And Tender Roast Turkey

I often buy the precooked, boneless roast turkey breast sold in 1-2 pound pieces in the grocery. This recipe gives it a little more home-cooked taste with almost no effort.

1 10¾-ounce can 97% fat-free cream of chicken soup
½ soup can water
1 2-pound precooked, fat-free, boneless roast turkey breast
   piece
No-stick cooking spray

Combine the soup and water. Slice the turkey breast into ¼" slices. Place the sliced turkey in a baking dish that has been coated with no-stick cooking spray. Pour the soup mixture over the turkey. Bake, covered, for 30 minutes at 350 degrees.

8 servings
3 fat grams per serving

Rich And Creamy Chicken Bake

1 10¾-ounce can 97% fat-free cream of mushroom soup
1-ounce package dehydrated onion soup mix
4 4-ounce chicken breast halves, skinned and boned
No-stick cooking spray

Combine the mushroom soup and dehydrated onion soup mix. Place the chicken breasts in a baking dish that has been coated with no-stick cooking spray. Spread the mixed soups over the chicken. Cover and bake for 30 minutes at 350 degrees.

4 servings
4 fat grams per serving

Roasted Deviled Chicken Breasts

1 tablespoon lemon juice
2 tablespoons liquid fat-free margarine
1 teaspoon prepared mustard
¼ teaspoon ground red pepper
1 teaspoon garlic powder
6 4-ounce chicken breasts halves, skinned and boned
No-stick cooking spray

Combine the lemon juice, liquid margarine, mustard, red pepper and garlic powder. Place the chicken breasts in a baking dish that has been coated with no-stick cooking spray. Brush the breasts with the basting mixture. Roast, covered, at 350 degrees for 20 minutes, or until juices run clear when pierced with a fork.

6 servings
4 fat grams per serving

Slow Cooker Mushroom Chicken

This recipe is so easy that you can decide to prepare it five minutes before you leave for work in the morning. It will cook by itself and be ready for you to serve by dinnertime.

4 4-ounce chicken breast halves, skinned and boned
1 8-ounce can sliced mushrooms, drained
1 10¾-ounce can 97% fat-free cream of chicken soup
Light salt and pepper to taste (optional)

Place the chicken in the slow cooker. Top with the mushrooms. Spread the chicken soup over all, adding light salt and pepper, if desired. Cook on low for 8-10 hours.

4 servings
5 fat grams per serving

Slow Cooker Cranberry Chicken

2 medium onions, cut into wedges
6 carrots, peeled and cut into 2" pieces
6 4-ounce chicken breasts, boned and skinned
1 15-ounce can whole berry cranberry sauce
½ cup fat-free French salad dressing
1 tablespoon lemon juice

Place the vegetables in the bottom of a slow cooker. Top with the chicken breasts. Combine the cranberry sauce and the French dressing. Pour the mixture over the chicken and vegetables. Cook on low for 8-10 hours.

6 servings
4 fat grams per serving

Spectacular Stuffed Chicken Breasts

A special dish that is good to serve to company. If you want to simplify, it is a good replacement for traditional turkey and stuffing at a holiday meal.

6 4-ounce chicken breast halves, boned and skinned
1 box cornbread stuffing mix, prepared according to package
    directions, omitting margarine
No-stick cooking spray
1 10¾-ounce can 97% fat-free cream of mushroom soup
½ cup water
1 8-ounce can sliced mushrooms, drained

Place each chicken breast between two sheets of waxed paper. Using a meat mallet or heavy, flat object, flatten the chicken. Place several tablespoons of the stuffing mixture on one side of each breast and roll up. Place seam side down in a baking dish that has been coated with no-stick cooking spray. Combine the mushroom soup, water and mushrooms. Pour the soup mixture over the chicken. Bake, covered, for 45 minutes at 350 degrees.

6 servings
5 fat grams per serving

Turkey Divan Casserole

Traditional Turkey Divan is made with whole spears of broccoli topped with sliced turkey and a rich, creamy sauce. I really like this version better. Of course, chicken can easily be substituted for the turkey.

3 cups cooked white rice
2 10-ounce boxes frozen, chopped broccoli, cooked
1 medium onion, finely chopped
2 cups cooked turkey breast, cubed
No-stick cooking spray
1 10¾-ounce can 97% fat-free cream of mushroom soup
1 cup fat-free sour cream
Light salt and pepper to taste (optional)

Combine the rice, broccoli, onion and turkey in a casserole dish that has been coated with no-stick cooking spray. Combine the soup and sour cream. Add the light salt and pepper to the soup mixture, if desired. Combine the soup with the rice mixture. Cover and bake for 30 minutes at 350 degrees.

6 servings
4 fat grams per serving

Uptown Chicken Hollandaise

Hollandaise sauce is probably the most lethal sauce in the world, since its main ingredients are melted butter and egg yolks. This dish is crowned with a fat-free version of Hollandaise that is still very good—yet totally healthy.

4 4-ounce chicken breast halves, skinned and boned
No-stick cooking spray
¾ cup fat-free mayonnaise
2 teaspoons lemon juice
¼ cup skim milk
4 English muffin halves, toasted

Sauté the chicken breasts in a skillet that has been coated with no-stick cooking spray for about 6 minutes per side. When they are browned and thoroughly cooked, remove them from the skillet. In a saucepan over low heat, combine the mayonnaise, lemon juice and skim milk. Place each chicken breast on a toasted English muffin half on a dinner plate. When the sauce is warm, spoon several tablespoons over each chicken breast.

4 servings
4 fat grams per serving

Pork Main Dishes

American Dinner Pie

The traditional English dish, Shepherd's Pie, contains beef and gravy topped with a blanket of mashed potatoes. This recipe uses the American favorites wieners and baked beans to create our own down home version.

1 pound fat-free wieners, cut into slices
2 15-ounce cans fat-free baked beans
1 medium onion, chopped
½ cup ketchup
No-stick cooking spray
2 cups prepared fat-free mashed potatoes
½ cup fat-free sour cream
1 cup fat-free Cheddar cheese

Combine the wieners, baked beans, onions and ketchup. Place in a baking dish that has been coated with no-stick cooking spray. Combine the mashed potatoes, sour cream and Cheddar cheese. Spread the potatoes over the bean mixture. Bake for 30 minutes at 350 degrees.

6 servings
0 fat grams per serving

Ashley's Chinese Burritos

My daughter Ashley has always enjoyed Mo Shu Pork in Chinese restaurants. The authentic version involves Chinese pancakes wrapped around a mixture of Chinese vegetables and meat. This is a quick and easy version to make at home using flour tortillas—a real international combination!

8 ounces pork tenderloin, all fat removed
No-stick cooking spray
2 cups cabbage, finely shredded
1 medium onion, thinly sliced
1 8-ounce can sliced mushrooms, drained
1 tablespoon light soy sauce
½ teaspoon Chinese sesame oil
1 13 ½-ounce package fat-free flour tortillas
1 cup fat-free barbecue sauce

Cut the pork tenderloin into matchstick-size pieces. Sauté in a skillet that has been coated with no-stick cooking spray. When the pork is lightly browned, remove from the skillet and sauté the cabbage and onions until tender-crisp. Return the pork to the skillet and add the mushrooms, soy sauce and sesame oil. Meanwhile, puncture the plastic bag containing the flour tortillas and microwave them on medium for about 1 minute, or until they are pliable. Brush each tortilla with barbecue sauce. Place several tablespoons of the pork and vegetable mixture on one side of each tortilla, then roll up. Serve immediately.

5 servings
1 fat gram per serving

Autumn Pork Tenderloin Dinner

Autumn and winter are perfect times to enjoy this flavorful recipe. It will warm the heart and soul on a cold evening.

4 3-ounce slices pork tenderloin, all fat removed
No-stick cooking spray
4 medium sweet potatoes, peeled and cut into 1" chunks
4 cooking apples, peeled and sliced
1 cup water
2 tablespoons soy sauce
1 tablespoon sugar

Place the pork slices between two pieces of waxed paper and flatten with a meat mallet or other flat, heavy object. Sauté the pork in a skillet that has been coated with no-stick cooking spray for 6 minutes per side. Arrange the pork slices, the sweet potatoes and the apples in a baking dish that has also been coated with no-stick cooking spray. Combine the water, soy sauce and sugar in a measuring cup. Pour over the pork and vegetables. Bake, covered, for 40 minutes at 350 degrees or until the sweet potatoes are tender.

4 servings
4 fat grams per serving

Baked Pork Supreme

I really like letting the oven do most of the work in this recipe. As you know, my motto is "make it simple, fix it quick and get out of the kitchen!"

4 3-ounce slices pork tenderloin, all fat removed
No-stick cooking spray
½ cup uncooked rice
1 medium onion, sliced
1 green pepper, sliced
1 15-ounce can tomatoes, chopped and drained (juice reserved)
Hot water
Light salt and pepper to taste (optional)

Place the pork slices between two pieces of waxed paper and flatten with a meat mallet or other heavy, flat object. Brown the slices on both sides over medium heat in a skillet that has been coated with no-stick cooking spray. Meanwhile, place the rice in a baking dish that has also been coated with no-stick cooking spray. Place the browned pork slices on the rice. Top each pork slice with onion and green pepper slices. Scatter the chopped tomatoes over the top. In a measuring cup, add enough hot water to the reserved tomato juice to equal 2 cups. Add light salt and pepper, if desired. Pour the water and tomato juice over the ingredients in the baking dish. Bake, tightly covered, at 350 degrees for 1 hour, or until the rice is tender.

4 servings
3 fat grams per serving

Busy Day Ham And Dumplings

I've had lots of positive comments about the chicken and dumplings recipe in *Live! Don't Diet!* This recipe uses the same surprise ingredient—flour tortillas. If you can't find the fat-free flour tortillas, most regular flour tortillas are still very low in fat and can be used.

6 cups water
1 ham or chicken bouillon cube
8 ounces 98% fat-free ham
1 13 ½-ounce package fat-free flour tortillas
1 10 ¾-ounce can 97% fat-free cream of mushroom soup
 (optional)
1 8-ounce can sliced mushrooms, drained (optional)

Combine the water, ham or chicken bouillon and ham in a medium saucepan. Bring to a boil over medium heat. Meanwhile cut the tortillas into 1" squares. Drop the tortilla squares slowly in to the boiling liquid. Stir frequently while adding the tortillas to keep them from sticking together. Lower the heat and simmer for about 15 minutes. Check frequently. When the dumplings are no longer doughy, add the mushroom soup and the mushrooms, if desired.

4 servings
2 fat grams per serving

Country-Style Pork Casserole

Sauerkraut seems to have a natural affinity for pork. The sweetness of the apples in this recipe mellows the usually sharp tang of the sauerkraut.

4 3-ounce slices pork tenderloin, all fat removed
No-stick cooking spray
2 cooking apples, peeled and sliced
1 medium onion, chopped
1 15-ounce can sauerkraut, drained
1 8-ounce can tomato sauce

Place the pork slices between two pieces of waxed paper and flatten with a meat mallet or other flat, heavy object. Sauté the pork in a skillet that has been coated with no-stick cooking spray for 6 minutes per side. In a mixing bowl, combine the apples, onion, sauerkraut and tomato sauce. Place the sauerkraut mixture in a casserole dish that has been coated with no-stick cooking spray. Place the pork on top of the sauerkraut. Bake, covered, for 40 minutes at 350 degrees.

4 servings
3 fat grams per serving

Creole Smoked Sausage

1 cup diced celery
1 medium bell pepper, coarsely chopped
1 medium onion, coarsely chopped
No-stick cooking spray
1 pound 97% fat-free smoked sausage, cut into 2" pieces
1 15-ounce can tomato sauce
1 15-ounce can tomatoes, chopped, with their juice
1 teaspoon garlic powder
Louisiana-style hot sauce to taste
1 tablespoon cornstarch

Sauté the celery, bell pepper and onion until tender in a skillet that has been coated with no-stick cooking spray. Remove the vegetables and sauté the sausage until lightly browned in the same skillet. Return the vegetables to the skillet. In a mixing bowl, combine the tomato sauce, tomatoes, garlic powder, hot sauce and cornstarch. Pour the sauce over the smoked sausage and vegetables in the skillet and simmer several minutes until the sauce has thickened.

4 servings
3 fat grams per serving

Deluxe Ham And Cheese Casserole

Who doesn't like ham and cheese? This recipe combines ham with two cheeses—and sour cream. Eating low-fat has never been better!

1 8-ounce can sliced mushrooms, drained
4 green onions, including tops, chopped
1 cup fat-free cottage cheese
1 cup fat-free sour cream
Light salt and pepper to taste (optional)
8 ounces 98% fat-free ham, cubed
1 cup fat-free Cheddar cheese, shredded
1 8-ounce package noodles, prepared according to
    package directions
No-stick cooking spray

Combine the mushrooms, green onions, cottage cheese, sour cream, light salt, pepper, ham, Cheddar cheese and noodles. Pour into a casserole dish that has been coated with no-stick cooking spray. Bake at 350 degrees. for 30 minutes.

4 servings
2 fat grams per serving

Deluxe Stuffed Wieners

This is an interesting and fun way to prepare wieners for a change. Great with slaw and baked beans.

1 package cornbread stuffing mix, prepared according to
    package directions, omitting margarine
1 pound fat-free wieners
5 tablespoons ketchup
No-stick cooking spray

Split each wiener almost in half lengthwise. Fill the split with several spoonfuls of the prepared stuffing. Top with ketchup. Bake for 20 minutes at 350 degrees.

5 servings
0 fat grams per serving

Extra-Lazy Sweet And Sour Ham

8 ounces precooked 98% fat-free ham, cut into matchstick-
    size pieces
1 large onion, cut into wedges
1 large bell pepper, cut into cubes
No-stick cooking spray
1 8-ounce can juice-packed pineapple tidbits
1 jar commercially-prepared, fat-free sweet and sour sauce
Hot, cooked rice

In a skillet that has been coated with no-stick cooking spray, sauté the ham, onion and bell pepper until the vegetables are tender-crisp. Add the pineapple and juice to the skillet, followed by the sweet and sour sauce. Simmer briefly. Serve over hot, cooked rice.

4 servings
1 fat gram per serving

Glorified Ham And Rice Casserole

2 cups cooked rice
2 10-ounce boxes frozen English peas, cooked according to
    package directions
8 ounces 98% fat-free ham, cubed
1 medium onion, coarsely chopped
1 teaspoon garlic powder
3 tablespoons fat-free grated Parmesan cheese
½ cup fat-free sour cream
½ cup fat-free mayonnaise
1 teaspoon lemon juice
Light salt and pepper to taste (optional)
No-stick cooking spray

Combine the rice, peas, ham and onion. In a separate mixing bowl, combine the garlic powder, Parmesan cheese, sour cream, mayonnaise, lemon juice. Add light salt and pepper to taste, if desired. Combine the sour cream mixture with the rice mixture. Place the mixture in a casserole dish that has been coated with no-stick cooking spray. Bake for 30 minutes at 350 degrees.

4 servings
2 fat grams per serving

Ham Casserole Deluxe

You probably wonder if we eat ham around my house every night, since I am including so many ham recipes. We really don't, but I do serve it often. I have always enjoyed ham, and since it is possible to buy it almost fat-free and precooked, it is a mainstay around my house for sandwiches, main courses and salads.

2 cups cooked rice
2 10-ounce packages chopped spinach, cooked and drained
1 medium onion, finely minced
1 8-ounce can sliced mushrooms, drained
8 ounces precooked 98% fat-free ham, diced
1 cup fat-free sour cream
¼ cup fat-free liquid margarine
1 1-ounce package dehydrated onion soup mix
Light salt and pepper to taste (optional)
No-stick cooking spray

Combine the rice, spinach, onion, mushrooms, ham, sour cream, liquid margarine, onion soup mix, light salt and pepper. Place the mixture in casserole dish that has been coated with no-stick cooking spray. Bake for 30 minutes at 350 degrees.

4 servings
2 fat grams per serving

Potato Stuffed Wieners

My mother made these for me as a child. I guess my inner child still loves them because I still like to make them. If you don't have leftover mashed potatoes, use instant mashed potatoes made according to package directions, omitting the margarine and using skim milk. Add 1 tablespoon fat-free sour cream to the potatoes. Use slightly less milk than the directions call for. The potatoes need to be fairly stiff.

1 cup leftover fat-free mashed potatoes
2 teaspoons dehydrated minced onion
¼ cup fat-free Cheddar cheese, shredded
1 pound fat-free wieners
No-stick cooking spray

Combine the mashed potatoes, onion and cheese. Cut each wiener almost in half lengthwise. Fill the slit in the wiener with about 2 tablespoons of the potato mixture. Place the wieners in a baking dish that has been coated with no-stick cooking spray. Bake for 20 minutes at 350 degrees.

5 servings
0 fat grams per serving

Red Beans And Rice Casserole

If you love the taste of red beans and rice, you'll like this casserole. Using canned beans may not be authentic, but it sure helps when you decide you would like to make this dish at the last minute.

4 cups cooked white rice
2 15-ounce cans red beans or kidney beans, rinsed and drained
1 medium onion, chopped
1 medium bell pepper, chopped
½ pound 97% fat-free smoked sausage, thinly sliced
1 15-ounce can chunky tomato sauce,
Light salt and pepper to taste (optional)
Louisiana hot sauce to taste
No-stick cooking spray

Combine the rice, beans, onion, bell pepper, smoked sausage, tomato sauce, light salt, pepper and hot sauce. Place in a casserole dish that has been coated with no-stick cooking spray. Bake, covered, for 1 hour at 350 degrees.

4 servings
1 fat gram per serving

Simple, Crispy Pork Cutlets

4 3-ounce slices pork tenderloin, all fat removed
¼ cup fat-free egg substitute
¼ cup water
1 teaspoon vegetable oil
1 cup cornflake crumbs
1 teaspoon garlic powder
Light salt and pepper to taste (optional)
No-stick cooking spray

Place the slices of pork between two sheets of waxed paper. Using a meat mallet or other heavy, flat object, flatten each slice. In a shallow dish, combine the egg substitute, water and oil. In another shallow dish, combine the cornflake crumbs and garlic powder. Add light salt and pepper, if desired. Dip each flattened slice of pork into the egg mixture, then into the crumbs. Place each coated slice in a baking dish that has been coated with no-stick cooking spray. Bake for 30 minutes or until browned at 400 degrees. Check frequently. Do not overcook.

4 servings
3 fat grams per serving

Slow Cooker New England-Style Dinner

This recipe replaces the corned beef in the traditional New England boiled dinner with ham and adds the convenience of slow cooking instead of boiling. The sauce may not exactly be traditional either, but it is good.

1 medium cabbage, cut into 4 large wedges
4 medium potatoes, peeled and cut into wedges
4 medium onions, peeled and cut into wedges
4 large carrots, scraped and cut into 2" pieces
4 4-ounce slices 98% fat-free ham
½ cup water

Sauce:
1 cup fat-free sour cream
2 tablespoons skim milk
Horseradish to taste

Place the cabbage, potatoes, onions and carrots in a slow cooker. Top with the ham slices. Pour the water over all and bake on low for 8-10 hours. Combine the sauce ingredients in a small saucepan and warm briefly. Serve along with the ham and vegetables.

4 servings
2 fat grams per serving

Smoked Sausage Italian-Style

My husband, Ken, has always loved Italian sausages cooked with peppers and onions. Since we began our low-fat lifestyle his favorite is a now much leaner variation.

1 pound 97% fat-free smoked sausage, sliced
No-stick cooking spray
1 medium onion, sliced
1 bell pepper, sliced

Sauté the sausage slices in a skillet that has been coated with no-stick cooking spray. When they are lightly brown, add the onions and pepper. Continue cooking until the vegetables are tender-crisp.

6 servings
1 fat gram per serving

Smoked Sausage Dinner In One Dish

1 pound 97% fat-free smoked sausage
3 medium potatoes, peeled and sliced
2 medium onions, chopped
4 carrots, scraped and cut into 2" pieces
15-ounce can chunky tomato sauce
No-stick cooking spray

Combine the smoked sausage, vegetables and tomato sauce in a casserole dish that has been coated with no-stick cooking spray. Bake, covered, for 45 minutes at 350 degrees, or until the vegetables are tender.

4 servings
2 fat grams per serving

Stick To Your Ribs Ham And Potatoes

2 cups instant potato flakes
2 cups boiling water
½ cup fat-free egg substitute
1 cup packaged seasoned, dry breadcrumbs
3 tablespoons dehydrated minced onion
Light salt and pepper to taste (optional)
No-stick cooking spray
8 ounces 98% fat-free precooked ham, diced
1 medium onion, chopped
1 10-ounce package frozen chopped broccoli, cooked and
    drained
1 cup fat-free sour cream

Combine the instant potato flakes and the boiling water. When cool, add the egg substitute, breadcrumbs, dehydrated minced onion and the light salt and pepper. Spread the mixture in a 8" x 8" baking dish that has been coated with no-stick cooking spray. Combine the ham, onion, broccoli and sour cream. Spread over the potato mixture. Bake for 30 minutes at 350 degrees.

4 servings
2 fat grams per serving

Stroganoff With Ham

When we think of stroganoff, we usually think of beef as the main ingredient. However, ham is a very good change of pace. Serve over rice or noodles.

1 pound fresh mushrooms, sliced
1 medium onion, sliced
No-stick cooking spray
8 ounces 98% fat-free ham, cut into matchstick-sized pieces
1 teaspoon garlic powder
1 cup fat-free sour cream
1 teaspoon Worcestershire sauce
Light salt and pepper to taste (optional)
1 8-ounce package noodles, prepared according to package
   directions

Sauté the mushrooms and onions in a skillet that has been coated with no-stick cooking spray. When they are tender, add the ham and continue cooking briefly. When the ham is slightly browned, add the garlic powder, sour cream, Worcestershire sauce and light salt and pepper, if desired. Serve on a bed of noodles or rice.

4 servings
3 fat grams per serving

Tempting Tenderloin Bake

It's hard to imagine life without pork. Thanks to pork tenderloin, we don't have to even think about doing without it. A 3-ounce serving of lean pork tenderloin has only 4 fat grams.

4 3-ounce slices pork tenderloin, all fat removed
No-stick cooking spray
1 medium onion, chopped
½ cup ketchup
¼ cup water
1 teaspoon garlic powder
3 tablespoons lemon juice
1 teaspoon dry mustard

Place the pork tenderloin slices between two sheets of waxed paper and flatten with a meat mallet or other flat, heavy object. Sauté the slices in a skillet that has been coated with no-stick cooking spray for 5 minutes per side or until lightly browned. Place the pork in a baking dish that has also been coated with no-stick cooking spray. Sprinkle the chopped onion over the pork. In a mixing bowl, combine the ketchup, water, garlic powder, lemon juice and dry mustard. Pour the sauce over the pork. Cover and bake for 30 minutes at 350 degrees.

4 servings
4 fat grams per serving

Seafood Main Dishes

Baked Fish In A Hurry

This is another one of those recipes that is great to make when preparation time is at a premium or when the pantry is almost bare—like mine becomes when I have put off going to the grocery store too many times.

6 4-ounce boneless perch or flounder fillets
1 10¾-ounce can 97% fat-free cream of mushroom soup
1 tablespoon dried parsley flakes
No-stick cooking spray

Place the fish in a baking dish that has been coated with no-stick cooking spray. Pour the soup over the fish and sprinkle with the parsley flakes. Cover and bake for 30 minutes at 350 degrees.

4 servings
3 fat grams per serving

Chinese-Style Sesame Shrimp

Stir-frying is a great way to cook. It doesn't take much oil and the ingredients retain their fresh texture and color. Those of us who want to get out of the kitchen fast love it because it is so quick—and doesn't mess up a lot of pots and pans!

1 tablespoon vegetable oil
No-stick cooking spray
1 pound fresh or thawed frozen shrimp, peeled and deveined
1 tablespoon sesame seeds
1 medium onion, cut into wedges
2 tablespoons reduced-sodium soy sauce
¼ teaspoon ground ginger
¼ teaspoon garlic powder
Hot, cooked rice

Add the oil to a wok or skill that has been coated with no-stick cooking spray. Heat the oil, then add the shrimp, onions, and sesame seeds. Cook over medium heat until the shrimp have turned pink. Do not overcook. Add the soy sauce, ginger and garlic powder. Serve with hot, cooked rice.

6 servings
5 fat grams per serving

Crispy Sesame Broiled Scallops

Scallops are the perfect seafood—no bones to worry about, like fish, no shells to peel off, like shrimp—just tender nuggets of wonderful flavor that cook in an instant.

1 pound scallops
1 tablespoon vegetable oil
½ cup commercially prepared seasoned dry breadcrumbs
1 tablespoon sesame seeds
Light salt and pepper to taste (optional)
No-stick cooking spray

Place the scallops and oil in a mixing bowl. Stir gently until all of the scallops are lightly coated. Drain off any excess oil. Place the breadcrumbs, sesame seeds, light salt and pepper in a zip-top plastic bag. Add the scallops a few at a time and shake gently to coat with the breadcrumb mixture. Place the scallops on a baking sheet that has been coated with no-stick cooking spray. Lightly coat the scallops with cooking spray. Broil 5" from the heat source for 3-4 minutes or until browned. Turn and broil for 3-4 more minutes. Watch carefully to prevent overcooking.

4 servings
8 fat grams per serving

Crunchy Tuna Casserole

Don't scream! Yes, I know you are probably not too excited about another tuna casserole recipe, but this one is different enough your family will love it.

2 8-ounce cans water-packed light chunk tuna
3 stalks celery, finely minced
1 medium onion, finely minced
1 8-ounce can sliced water chestnuts, drained
1 cup herb seasoned stuffing mix
1 cup fat-free mayonnaise
½ cup fat-free sour cream
2 tablespoons lemon juice
1 cup fat-free Cheddar cheese, shredded
Light salt and pepper to taste (optional)
No-stick cooking spray

Combine the tuna, celery, onion, water chestnuts, stuffing mix, mayonnaise, sour cream, lemon juice, cheese, salt and pepper in a baking dish that has been coated with no-stick cooking spray. Bake for 30 minutes at 350 degrees.

6 servings
1 fat gram per serving

Mandarin-Style Baked Snapper Fillets

Other low-fat fish fillets can be substituted for the snapper, if desired.

4 6-ounce snapper fillets
No-stick cooking spray
1 teaspoon vegetable oil
3 tablespoons water
1 tablespoon cornstarch
3 tablespoons reduced-sodium soy sauce
1 tablespoon vinegar
1 8-ounce can sliced water chestnuts, drained
Sugar substitute to equal 2 tablespoons sugar

Place the fillets in a baking dish that has been coated with no-stick cooking spray. Brush the fish lightly with oil and bake for 20 minutes at 350 degrees or until it flakes easily with a fork. Meanwhile, combine the water and cornstarch in a saucepan. Add the soy sauce, vinegar and water chestnuts. Bring to a boil, reduce the heat and simmer until thickened. Remove from the heat and add the sugar substitute. When the fish is done, remove to individual plates and top with the sauce.

4 servings
3 fat grams per serving

Oven-Baked Shrimp Jambalaya Casserole

This recipe combines some of the great spicy flavors that make it easy to eat low-fat. Louisiana hot sauce has become a mainstay around our house. It can add zip to just about anything. I even heard that there are folks who put it on ice cream!

1 pound salad-size frozen shrimp, thawed
3 cups cooked white rice
1 12-ounce package frozen sliced okra, thawed
1 15-ounce can tomatoes, chopped
1 8-ounce can tomato sauce
6 green onions, including tops, chopped
Light salt and pepper to taste (optional)
Red pepper to taste
1 teaspoon garlic powder
Louisiana hot sauce to taste
No-stick cooking spray

Combine the shrimp, rice, okra, tomatoes, tomato sauce, green onions, light salt and pepper, red pepper, garlic powder. and hot sauce. Place the mixture in a baking dish that has been coated with no-stick cooking spray. Bake for 30 minutes at 350 degrees or until the shrimp are pink.

6 servings
2 fat grams per serving

Oven-Fried Fish With Creamy Garlic Butter Sauce

4 6-ounce boneless perch or flounder fillets
1 tablespoon vegetable oil
1 cup cornflake crumbs
Light salt and pepper to taste (optional)
No-stick cooking spray

Sauce:
1 cup fat-free sour cream
¼ cup liquid fat-free margarine
1 teaspoon garlic powder
Light salt and pepper to taste (optional)
1 teaspoon dried parsley flakes

Lightly brush each fillet on both sides with oil. Combine the cornflake crumbs with the light salt and pepper to taste. Roll each fillet in the crumbs to coat. Place the fillets on a baking sheet that has been coated with no-stick cooking spray. Lightly spray the fillets with the cooking spray. Bake for 20 minutes at 425 degrees. Turn and bake for 10 minutes or until the fillets are browned and flake easily with a fork. Combine the sauce ingredients in a saucepan. Place over low heat, stirring frequently. When the sauce is warm, spoon over the fillets.

4 servings
2 fat grams per serving

Quick And Spicy Fish Fillets

One of the best parts of shrimp cocktail is the tangy horseradish-flavored cocktail sauce that usually accompanies it. This basic sauce adds it's own special zip to baked fish as well.

4 6-ounce perch or flounder fillets
No-stick cooking spray
1 15-ounce can tomato sauce
1 tablespoon horseradish (or to taste)
1 tablespoon lemon juice
1 teaspoon Worcestershire sauce

Place the fish fillets in a baking dish that has been coated with no-stick cooking spray. Combine the tomato sauce, horseradish, lemon juice and Worcestershire sauce. Pour over the fish and bake, covered, for 30 minutes at 350 degrees. The fish is done when it flakes easily with a fork.

4 servings
2 fat grams per serving

Saucy Shrimp And Pasta Au Gratin

Surprisingly, many brands of packaged macaroni and cheese are low in fat. Buy one of the low-fat brands and omit the butter and whole milk.

1 box low-fat macaroni and cheese (with powdered cheese
    sauce packet)
½ cup fat-free sour cream
1 teaspoon garlic powder
2 tablespoons dehydrated onion flakes
½ teaspoon red pepper
Light salt to taste
1 cup fat-free Cheddar cheese, shredded
1 cup cooked fresh or frozen shrimp or 1 8-ounce can shrimp
2 ounces precooked 98% fat-free ham finely minced
No-stick cooking spray

Cook the macaroni according to package directions. Drain the macaroni but allow several tablespoons of water to remain. Slowly add the powdered cheese sauce that comes with the boxed mix, stirring constantly to prevent lumps. Add the sour cream, garlic powder, onion flakes, red pepper, light salt and shredded Cheddar cheese. Add the shrimp and ham and combine thoroughly. Pour the mixture into a baking dish that has been coated with no-stick cooking spray. Bake for 30 minutes at 325 degrees.

4 servings
2 fat grams per serving

Scallop Sauté

Scallops are my favorite seafood. They are bite-size, mild in flavor and are relatively inexpensive compared to other shell-fish, at least in most parts of the country. They are also just plain good!

1 pound scallops
3 tablespoons lemon juice
1 teaspoon garlic powder
1 teaspoon dried parsley flakes
1 teaspoon vegetable oil
No-stick cooking spray

Combine the scallops, lemon juice, garlic powder and parsley flakes. Add the vegetable oil to a skillet that has been coated with no-stick cooking spray. Sauté the scallops over medium heat for 5-7 minutes or until they are lightly browned.

4 servings
2 fat grams per serving

Shrimp Stroganoff

I never get tired of the rich taste of stroganoff sauce but just in case you do, the addition of tomato sauce gives this dish a little different taste.

1 pound fresh shrimp or thawed frozen shrimp, peeled and deveined
No-stick cooking spray
1 15-ounce can tomato sauce
1 cup fat-free sour cream
2 tablespoons dehydrated minced onion
1 8-ounce can sliced mushrooms, drained
Light salt and pepper to taste (optional)
Hot, cooked rice

Sauté the shrimp in a skillet that has been coated with no-stick cooking spray for about 3 minutes or until pink. Do not overcook. Add the tomato sauce, sour cream, onion, mushrooms, light salt and pepper. Simmer briefly until warmed through. Serve over hot, cooked rice.

4 servings
3 fat grams per serving

Sunday Salmon Loaf

Read labels carefully when buying canned salmon. Some brands are quite high in fat, while others are much lower.

1 16-ounce can skinless, boneless pink salmon, flaked
1 cup soft bread crumbs, made from reduced-calorie bread
1 ½ cups skim milk
½ cup fat-free egg substitute
¼ cup liquid fat-free margarine
Light salt and pepper to taste (optional)
No-stick cooking spray

Combine the salmon and the bread crumbs. Add the milk, egg substitute, liquid fat-free margarine, light salt and pepper. Combine thoroughly. Place the mixture in a 9" x 5" loaf pan. Bake for 1 hour at 350 degrees.

4 servings
4 fat grams per serving

Tempting Baked Fish

1 cup fat-free sour cream
1 tablespoon prepared mustard
1 teaspoon dehydrated onion flakes
4 6-ounce perch or flounder fillets
1 cup dry breadcrumbs
No-stick cooking spray

Combine the sour cream, mustard and onion flakes. Spread both sides of each fish fillet with the mixture, then coat with the breadcrumbs. Place the coated fillets in a baking dish that has been coated with no-stick cooking spray. Bake for 20 minutes at 400 degrees or until the fish is lightly browned and flakes easily with a fork.

4 servings
3 fat grams per serving

Tuna-Rice Casserole

This is a versatile recipe. If you are not in the mood for tuna, chicken breast or low-fat ham works equally well.

3 cups cooked white rice
1 8-ounce can water-packed light tuna, drained and flaked
1 cup fat-free sour cream
¼ cup liquid fat-free margarine
1 1-ounce package dehydrated onion soup mix
1 medium onion, finely minced
Pepper to taste (optional)
No-stick cooking spray

Combine the rice, tuna, sour cream, margarine, onion soup mix, onion and pepper. Place the mixture in a baking dish that has been coated with no-stick cooking spray. Bake for 30 minutes at 350 degrees.

4 servings
1 fat gram per serving

Zesty Fish Scampi

Shrimp Scampi is a flavorful dish found on the menu of many seafood restaurants. While it is a delicious way to prepare shrimp, even at home, there are times when we don't really want to blow the grocery budget on shrimp. Using a mild, low-fat fish can provide the flavor without the cost.

4 4-ounce fillets of your favorite mild, low-fat fish
No-stick cooking spray
½ cup fat-free Italian salad dressing
½ teaspoon coarsely ground black pepper
1 teaspoon dried parsley flakes

Place the fillets in a baking dish that has been coated with no-stick cooking spray. Combine the Italian dressing, pepper and parsley flakes. Pour over the fish. Cover and bake for 30 minutes at 325 degrees. The fish will be done when it flakes easily with a fork.

4 servings
Fat grams per serving will vary depending on fish used.
The sauce contains no fat

Meatless Main Dishes

Baked Egg Foo Young

I used to love ordering Egg Foo Young in Chinese restaurants but those delicious patties soak up oil like a sponge. The baked version is fat-free and infinitely better for you.

1 large onion, finely chopped
1 large bell pepper, finely chopped
No-stick cooking spray
1 15-ounce can bamboo shoots, drained
2 cups fat-free egg substitute
1 tablespoon cornstarch
Light salt and pepper to taste (optional)

Sauce:
1 10½-ounce can low-fat beef gravy
1 tablespoon low-sodium soy sauce

Sauté the onion and pepper in a skillet that has been coated with no-stick cooking spray. When tender, add the bean sprouts and continue cooking 5 minutes. Remove the vegetables from the heat and allow them to cool. Meanwhile, in a mixing bowl, combine the egg substitute, cornstarch, salt and pepper. Add the cooled vegetables to the egg mixture. Pour into a baking dish that has been coated with no-stick cooking spray. Bake for 30 minutes at 350 degrees or until a knife inserted into the center comes out clean. In a saucepan, combine the sauce ingredients and heat until warm. To serve, cut the Egg Foo Young into 4 servings and place one on each dinner plate. Top with a portion of the sauce.

4 servings
1 fat gram per serving

Baked Lasagna With Cream Sauce

Traditional lasagna with hearty tomato sauce is great but this version with cream sauce is just as tasty and satisfying.

2 cups skim milk
½ cup fat-free sour cream
4 tablespoons cornstarch
Light salt and pepper to taste (optional)
1 10-ounce package frozen chopped spinach, cooked and
  squeezed dry
2 cups fat-free cottage cheese
1 cup fat-free mozzarella, shredded
¼ cup fat-free Parmesan cheese, grated
1 tablespoon garlic powder
¼ cup fat-free egg substitute
1 8-ounce package lasagna noodles, cooked according to
  package directions
No-stick cooking spray

Combine the milk, sour cream, cornstarch, light salt and pepper. Place in a saucepan and cook over low heat, stirring often, until thickened. In a mixing bowl, combine the spinach, cottage cheese, mozzarella cheese, Parmesan cheese, garlic powder and egg substitute. In a 9" x 13" baking dish that has been coated with no-stick cooking spray, spread a thin layer of the cream sauce. Top with 3 of the cooked lasagna noodles, followed by ⅓ of the sauce and ½ of the cheese mixture. Top the cheese mixture with 3 more noodles, ⅓ cup of the cream sauce, the remaining cheese mixture and the last 3 noodles. Spread the final ⅓ of the cream sauce on top. Cover with foil and bake for 30 minutes at 350 degrees. Let stand 10 minutes.

8 servings
1 fat gram per serving

Creamy Fettucini

This recipe is a country cousin of that rich Italian specialty Fettuccini Alfredo. Serve with a mixed green salad and Italian bread.

16-ounce package fettuccini noodles, cooked according to
    package directions
1 15-ounce can sliced mushrooms, drained
1 15-ounce can tomatoes, chopped and drained
1 cup fat-free sour cream
¼ cup liquid fat-free margarine
½ cup fat-free grated Parmesan cheese
1 teaspoon garlic powder
1 tablespoon lemon juice
Light salt and pepper to taste (optional)
1 tablespoon dried parsley flakes

In a saucepan, combine the cooked noodles, mushrooms, chopped tomatoes, sour cream, liquid margarine, Parmesan cheese, garlic powder, lemon juice, light salt and pepper and parsley flakes. Simmer briefly until heated through. Top with additional Parmesan cheese if desired.

4 servings
1 fat gram per serving

Easy Cheesy Pie

Not only is this savory pie easy to put together, it also makes its own crust. The crust does best if you use a glass pie plate instead of a metal one.

2 cups fat-free Cheddar cheese, shredded
1 medium onion, chopped
1 8-ounce can sliced mushrooms, drained
No-stick cooking spray
2 cups skim milk
1 cup fat-free egg substitute
½ teaspoon red pepper
Light salt and pepper to taste (optional)
½ cup all-purpose flour
2 teaspoons baking powder

Combine the cheese, onion and mushrooms in a pie plate that has been coated with no-stick cooking spray. Combine the milk, egg substitute, red pepper, light salt, pepper, flour and baking powder and stir until well blended. Pour the milk mixture over the cheese and vegetables. Bake for 45 minutes at 350 degrees. The pie will be done when a knife inserted into the center comes out clean.

4 servings
0 fat grams per serving

Old-Fashioned Potato Dumplings

I have heard older people reminiscing about eating potato dumplings during the Great Depression. They were popular because they were inexpensive, yet very filling and very good. That's still the reason to enjoy them today. Canned or homemade chicken broth can be used in place of the water and bouillon. Just make sure it is low-fat.

4 large baking potatoes, peeled and cubed
6 cups water
2 packets chicken or ham bouillon, low-sodium if possible
1 13 ½-ounce package flour tortillas, cut into 1" squares
1 10 ¾-ounce can 97% fat-free cream of mushroom soup
½ cup fat-free sour cream
Light salt and pepper to taste (optional)

Place the potatoes, water and bouillon in a saucepan over medium heat. Bring to a boil, reduce the heat, cover and let simmer for about 30 minutes or until the potatoes are easily pierced with a knife. When the potatoes are tender, slowly add the tortilla squares a few at the time, stirring frequently. Add additional water if needed. Simmer for approximately 10 minutes or until the dumplings are tender. Add the mushroom soup, sour cream, light salt and pepper to taste (optional).

4 servings
1 fat gram per serving

Rich Ravioli Casserole

This is so quick and easy that it is almost embarrassing. As I mentioned in a previous recipe, one of the most popular national brands of cheese ravioli is now fat-free. As long as the public continues to demand it, companies will continue to reduce the fat in popular commercially prepared foods. That is a real blessing to those of us who love to eat but don't want the fat.

2 15-ounce cans fat-free cheese ravioli
No-stick cooking spray
2 cups fat-free cottage cheese
¼ cup fat-free Parmesan cheese, grated
1 cup fat-free mozzarella
¼ cup fat-free egg substitute
1 10-ounce package frozen spinach, cooked and squeezed dry
Light salt and pepper to taste (optional)

Layer 1 can of the cheese ravioli in a baking dish that has been coated with no-stick cooking spray. Combine the cottage cheese, Parmesan cheese, mozzarella cheese, egg substitute, spinach, light salt and pepper. Spread over the ravioli. Spoon the contents of the remaining can of ravioli over the cheese layer. Cover tightly with aluminum foil and bake for 30 minutes at 350 degrees. Uncover and bake for 10 more minutes. Allow to stand for about 10 minutes before serving. Sprinkle with additional fat-free Parmesan cheese if desired.

4 servings
0 fat grams per serving

Shortcut Lasagna

With this easy recipe, the noodles don't have to be boiled. Homemade lasagna can be ready for the oven in minutes.

1 large onion, chopped
No-stick cooking spray
1 tablespoon garlic powder, divided
2 15-ounce cans tomato sauce
1 cup water
1 15-ounce can sliced mushrooms, drained
1 tablespoon dried oregano
2 cups fat-free cottage cheese
1 cup fat-free mozzarella shredded
¼ cup fat-free Parmesan cheese, grated
¼ cup fat-free egg substitute
Light salt and pepper to taste
8-ounce package lasagna noodles, uncooked

Sauté the onion in a saucepan that has been coated with no-stick cooking spray. Add 2 teaspoons of the garlic powder, the tomato sauce, water, mushrooms and the oregano. In a mixing bowl, combine the remaining 1 teaspoon garlic powder, the cottage cheese, mozzarella, Parmesan cheese and the egg substitute. Add light salt and pepper to taste (optional).

In a 9" x 11" baking dish that has been coated with no-stick cooking spray, spread 1 cup of the sauce. Top with three uncooked noodles followed by half of the cheese mixture. Spread 1 cup sauce on top of the cheese mixture. Add three more noodles, followed by the remaining cheese mixture, 1 cup sauce, the remaining three noodles and the remaining sauce. Sprinkle with additional grated Parmesan if desired. Cover tightly with foil and bake for 45 minutes at 350 degrees. Uncover and bake for 15 additional minutes. Allow to stand for 10-15 minutes.

8 servings
1 fat gram per serving

South Of The Border Baked Tacos

These are tacos without the mess. Since the tacos are baked in a casserole, they are eaten with a fork. Therefore, the filling ends up in our mouths instead of our laps! Add a bit of low-fat browned ground round or chopped chicken breast to the filling if you wish.

12 fat-free corn tortillas
1 15-ounce can fat-free or low-fat refried beans
2 cups fat-free Cheddar cheese, shredded
2 cups fat-free cottage cheese
1 medium onion, finely chopped
2 15-ounce cans chunky taco sauce

Toppings:
Finely shredded lettuce
Fat-free shredded Cheddar cheese
Fat-free sour cream
Hot or mild taco sauce
Finely chopped onion

Soften the tortillas by puncturing the package and microwaving them for 30 seconds. Spread about 2 tablespoons of the refried beans down the center of each tortilla. Combine the Cheddar cheese, cottage cheese and chopped onion. Place a generous amount down the center of each tortilla. Enclose the filling by folding both sides of the tortilla to the center. Spread a thin layer of taco sauce in a 9" x 13" baking dish that has been coated with no-stick cooking spray. Lay each stuffed tortilla seam side down in the baking dish. Pour the remaining sauce over the tacos. Cover tightly with aluminum foil and bake for 30 minutes at 350 degrees. Just before serving add the toppings or allow each person to add their own at the table.

4 servings
0 fat grams per taco

Terrific Enchiladas

Don't laugh! Potatoes make a hearty and rich filling for enchiladas. I give potatoes a lot of the credit for my weight loss. I love them any way they are prepared. Being able to enjoy a hot baked potato, oven fries or a rich potato casserole prepared with low-fat ingredients is so satisfying. It is definitely not deprivation.

12 fat-free corn tortillas (1 package)
2 cups fat-free mashed potatoes (see recipe index)
1 ½ cups fat-free Cheddar cheese, divided
½ cup fat-free cottage cheese
1 medium onion, chopped
¼ cup fat-free egg substitute
Light salt and pepper to taste (optional)
2 15-ounce cans chunky Mexican-style tomato sauce
No-stick cooking spray

Punch several holes in the tortilla package and microwave 30 seconds to soften them. Combine the mashed potatoes, 1 cup of the Cheddar cheese, the cottage cheese, onion, egg substitute, light salt and pepper. Spread a thin layer of the tomato sauce in a 9" x 13" baking dish that has been coated with no-stick cooking spray. Remove a warm tortilla from the package and place several tablespoons of the mashed potato filling down the center of each tortilla. Fold both sides to the middle. Place seam side down in the baking dish. Continue filling all of the tortillas. Cover the filled tortillas with the tomato sauce. Cover tightly with foil and bake for 30 minutes at 350 degrees. Allow to stand several minutes before serving. Just before serving, top with the remaining ½ cup cheese.

4 servings
0 fat grams per serving

Breads

Apple Fritters

Fritters are a beloved staple of the American kitchen. Unfortunately, they are also fried, so they are loaded with fat. A fritter can absorb up to a tablespoon of oil in the frying process. So, we simply bake our fritters instead of frying them. "But isn't that just a muffin?" you ask. No, a fritter has a heavier, chewier texture than a muffin. That's part of what makes it so satisfying.

¼ cup egg substitute
1 cup skim milk
¼ cup unsweetened applesauce
2 tablespoons sugar and 3 packets sugar substitute
¼ teaspoon light salt
3 cups all-purpose flour
2 teaspoons baking powder
¼ teaspoon nutmeg
¼ teaspoon cinnamon
1 ½ cups apple, peeled and coarsely chopped
No-stick cooking spray

Combine the egg substitute, skim milk, and applesauce. Add the sugar, salt, flour, baking powder, nutmeg and cinnamon. Stir just until the ingredients are combined, then fold in the chopped apple. Spoon into miniature muffin tins that have been coated with no-stick cooking spray. Bake for 20 minutes at 350 degrees. For an added treat, serve with apple butter.

24 fritters
0 fat grams per fritter

Baked Banana Fritters

Here is another baked fritter recipe. I used to love to dine at luau-style restaurants. They might have been hokey to the sophistocated crowd, but I thought they were loads of fun. Many of them served only a few desserts and one of them was usually fried bananas. They were actually batter dipped chunks of fruit that resembled fritters. There aren't many of these restaurants around now but I can make my own version of those fritters at home.

¼ cup egg substitute
1 cup skim milk
¼ cup fat-free sour cream
¼ cup sugar
¼ teaspoon light salt
3 cups all-purpose flour
2 teaspoons baking powder
¼ teaspoon nutmeg
¼ teaspoon cinnamon
2 medium bananas, very coarsely chopped
No-stick cooking spray

Combine the egg substitute and skim milk. Add the sour cream, sugar, salt, flour, baking powder, nutmeg and cinnamon. Stir just until all ingredients are combined. Add the chopped bananas and stir them into the batter. Spoon into miniature muffin tins that have been coated with no-stick cooking spray. Bake for 25 minutes at 350 degrees.

24 fritters
0 fat grams per fritter

Blueberry Bran Muffins

It is widely recognized that wheat bran is very good for you. It can also be very tasty when added to muffins or other breads. This is a delicious way to add fiber to your food.

1 ½ cups bran cereal
½ cup boiling water
1 ⅓ cups whole wheat flour
1 ¼ teaspoons baking soda
⅓ cup sugar or ¼ cup sugar and 2 packets sugar substitute
½ teaspoon cinnamon
¼ teaspoon nutmeg
¼ cup fat-free egg substitute
½ cup fat-free sour cream
¾ cup fresh or frozen blueberries
No-stick cooking spray

Combine the bran cereal and boiling water and let stand 15 minutes. Combine the flour, baking soda, sugar and spices. Add the cereal, then the egg substitute, and sour cream. Stir just until ingredients are combined. Fold in the blueberries. Spoon into muffin tins that have been coated with no-stick cooking spray. Bake for 25 minutes at 350 degrees.

12 muffins
0 fat grams per muffin

Classic Corn Fritters

1 15-ounce can creamed corn
3 tablespoons finely minced onion
½ cup fat-free egg substitute
1 cup self-rising flour
½ teaspoon light salt
No-stick cooking spray

Combine the corn, onion and egg substitute. Gradually add the flour and salt. Spoon into miniature muffin tins that have been coated with no-stick cooking spray. Bake for 30 minutes at 350 degrees.

24 fritters
0 fat grams per fritter

Classic Muffins

2 cups all-purpose flour
2 tablespoons sugar and 3 packets sugar substitute
¼ cup fat-free egg substitute
1 ½ cups skim milk
3 tablespoons applesauce
No-stick cooking spray

Combine the dry ingredients. Add the egg substitute, milk and applesauce. Stir until the ingredients are just combined. Spoon into muffin tins that have been coated with no-stick cooking spray. Bake for 25 minutes at 375 degrees. Variation: Add ½ cup blueberries or finely chopped apple.

12 muffins
0 fat grams per muffin

Comforting Cornbread

This recipe makes a moist, delicious cornbread. I love cornbread because it is filling and goes so well with soups and the homestyle dishes that we eat at our house. It is one of my comfort foods. I think that it is important to learn how to prepare our favorite comfort foods in a low-fat way. The foods that we have emotional ties to are those that we often turn to when we are stressed or tired or just plain hungry. They make us feel better. Having to give up some of my comfort foods is one of the reasons diets never worked for me. Thank goodness I finally learned that I really didn't have to give them up to lose.

1 cup self-rising cornmeal
1 ½ cups water
½ cup fat-free egg substitute
No-stick cooking spray

Preheat your oven to 400 degrees. Combine the dry ingredients. Slowly add the water while stirring constantly. Add the egg substitute. Pour the mixture into an 8" iron skillet or 8" square baking pan that has been coated with no-stick cooking spray. Bake for 30 minutes or until brown.

Variation: Add 2 tablespoons imitation bacon bits, 2 tablespoons minced dried onion and ½ cup shredded fat-free Cheddar cheese. Finely minced hot pepper or red pepper flakes may be added.

4 servings
1 fat gram per serving

Kind Of Donuts

These morsels are reminiscent of one of my favorite goodies— cake donuts. They are close enough in taste to satisfy that donut craving, without the fat!

1 ½ cups all-purpose flour
1 ½ teaspoons baking powder
⅓ cup sugar
¼ teaspoon light salt
¼ teaspoon nutmeg
½ cup skim milk
¼ cup fat-free egg substitute
No-stick cooking spray
10 packets aspartame-based sugar substitute
1 teaspoon cinnamon

Combine the flour, baking powder, sugar, salt and nutmeg. Gradually add the milk and the egg substitute. Spoon the mixture into mini-muffin tins that have been coated with no-stick cooking spray. Bake for 20 minutes at 350 degrees. When they are done, turn out onto a plate to cool. When they are cool, spray each muffin lightly with no-stick cooking spray. Combine the sugar substitute and cinnamon. Place the mixture in a zip-top plastic bag. Place the muffins in the bag and toss to coat with the mixture.

24 muffins
0 fat grams per muffin

Lazy Day Apple Muffins

This recipe is so easy that it is almost not a recipe at all! Try it when you are in a real hurry—or on those days when you want something warm and comforting to eat, but can't face more than a few minutes in the kitchen.

1 box low-fat yellow cake mix
½ cup fat-free egg substitute
1 cup water
1 15-ounce can unsweetened sliced apples, coarsely chopped
1 teaspoon nutmeg
No-stick cooking spray

Combine the cake mix, egg substitute and water. Fold in the apples and nutmeg. Spoon into muffin tins that have been coated with no-stick cooking spray. Bake for 30 minutes at 350 degrees.

12 muffins
1 fat gram per muffin

Mom's Yeast Cornbread

Another cornbread variation that is nice for a change. The yeast adds volume, as well as a lovely aroma and taste. I can never smell yeast without becoming ravenously hungry. Thank goodness many yeast breads are low in fat, so I don't have to feel guilty about indulging my love for them.

1 ½ cups plain cornmeal
¾ cup flour
1 ½ teaspoons baking powder
1 teaspoon salt
½ teaspoon baking soda
1 tablespoon sugar
1 package dry yeast
¾ cup fat-free egg substitute
2 cups low-fat buttermilk
No-stick cooking spray

Combine the dry ingredients. Add the egg substitute and the buttermilk. Pour into an iron skillet or baking pan that has been coated with no-stick cooking spray. Bake for 30 minutes at 425 degrees.

6 servings
1 fat gram per serving

Onion Flatbread

I love cooked onions. There is something so elemental, yet luxurious about them. Even when sautéed without oil, they become caramelized and develop a richness that we usually associate with cooking in lots of butter or oil. Combine that flavor with the wonderful taste of yeast bread and you have a really great treat.

2 large onions, thinly sliced
Butter-flavored no-stick cooking spray
¼ teaspoon garlic powder
Light salt and pepper to taste
1 loaf frozen white bread dough, thawed

Sauté the onions in a skillet that has been coated with no-stick cooking spray. When they become a rich caramel brown, add the garlic powder and light salt and pepper to taste. Meanwhile, press the thawed bread dough into a 9" x 13" baking dish that has been coated with no-stick cooking spray. Spread the onions over the dough. Lightly coat the surface with the no-stick cooking spray. Bake for 30 minutes at 350 degrees.

12 servings
0 fat grams per serving

Poor Folks' Pizza

This isn't really pizza, of course. I just jokingly call it that because it sort of resembles slices of pizza. My husband, Ken and I love cornbread and eat it often. We eat it so often, in fact, that one night I decided to serve it a little differently, for variety. I split each wedge in half horizontally and topped each piece with liquid fat-free margarine, finely chopped mild onion and shredded fat-free Cheddar cheese.

1 cup self-rising cornmeal mix
1 cup water
¼ cup fat-free egg substitute
2 tablespoons fat-free sour cream
No-stick cooking spray

Toppings:
Liquid fat-free margarine or ketchup
Finely chopped mild onion
Fat-free Cheddar cheese, shredded

Slowly add the water to the cornmeal mix. Add the egg substitute and sour cream. Pour into an 8" iron skillet or baking pan that has been coated with no-stick cooking spray. Bake for 30 minutes at 400 degrees or until brown and crusty. Cut into 6 pie-shaped wedges. Cut each wedge in half horizontally. Top with margarine or ketchup, followed by finely chopped onion and cheese. Serve immediately.

4 servings
1 fat gram per serving

Quick Apple-Cinnamon Muffins

¾ cup low-fat baking mix
1 envelope instant apple cinnamon oatmeal
½ cup skim milk
¼ cup fat-free egg substitute
No-stick cooking spray

Combine the baking mix and instant oatmeal. Add the skim milk and egg substitute. Spoon into 6 muffin cups that have been coated with no-stick cooking spray. Bake for 15 minutes at 375 degrees.

6 muffins
0 fat grams per muffin

Sweet Potato Muffins

½ cup fat-free egg substitute
1 cup skim milk
1 cup cooked, mashed sweet potatoes (fresh or canned)
⅓ cup unsweetened applesauce
1 ½ cups all-purpose flour
1 tablespoon sugar
5 teaspoons baking powder
½ teaspoon salt
½ teaspoon nutmeg
No-stick cooking spray

Combine the egg substitute, skim milk, sweet potatoes and applesauce. Mix until smooth. In a separate bowl, combine the dry ingredients. Add the dry ingredients to the potato mixture and stir just until combined. Spoon into muffin tins that have been coated with no-stick cooking spray. Each muffin cup should be ⅔ full. Bake for 30 minutes at 375 degrees.

12 muffins
0 fat grams per muffin

Vegetables

Coffee Baked Beans

2 15-ounce cans fat-free baked beans, drained
1 medium onion, finely minced
2 tablespoons ketchup
2 teaspoons prepared mustard
1 tablespoon Worcestershire sauce
3 packets sugar substitute
1 teaspoon instant coffee granules

Combine the beans, onion, ketchup, mustard, Worcestershire sauce, sugar substitute and coffee granules in a microwave-proof baking dish. Mix well. Cover and microwave on medium power for 10 minutes. Stir before serving.

8 servings
0 fat grams per serving

My Mom's Broccoli Casserole

2 10-ounce packages frozen broccoli, cooked and drained
I medium onion, finely minced
1 cup fat-free mayonnaise
½ cup fat-free egg substitute
4 tablespoons fat-free liquid margarine
1 can 97% fat-free cream of mushroom soup
1 cup fat-free Cheddar cheese, shredded
Light salt and pepper to taste (optional)
No-stick cooking spray

Combine all of the ingredients. Pour into a casserole dish that has been coated with no-stick cooking spray. Bake for 30 minutes at 350 degrees.

8 servings
1 fat gram per serving

Sautéed Broccoli Oriental

3 large stalks broccoli
no-stick cooking spray
2 tablespoons low-sodium soy sauce
1 teaspoon garlic powder

Wash the broccoli, peel the tough lower stems and chop into bite-sized pieces. Sauté the broccoli in a skillet that has been coated with no-stick cooking spray. When it is tender-crisp, add the soy sauce and garlic powder. Cover and steam for 2-3 minutes.

4 servings
0 fat grams per serving

The Best Brussels Sprouts

Brussels sprouts have long been considered bad news by children and by some adults too. Like spinach, they suffer from undeserved jokes about their taste. They are really good.

2 10-ounce packages frozen Brussels sprouts
2 tablespoons liquid fat-free margarine
1 tablespoon lemon juice
1 teaspoon Worcestershire sauce
Light salt and pepper to taste (optional)

In a saucepan over medium heat, bring 5 cups water to a boil. Add the sprouts and cook for approximately 10 minutes, or until tender. Drain the water and add the margarine, lemon juice and Worcestershire sauce. Add light salt and pepper to taste if desired.

4 servings
0 fat grams per serving

Skillet Cabbage Supreme

1 medium head cabbage, coarsely chopped
1 medium onion, coarsely chopped
1 medium bell pepper, coarsely chopped
2 stalks celery, coarsely chopped
No-stick cooking spray
1 tablespoon imitation bacon bits
1 15-ounce can tomato sauce
2 packets sugar substitute

Sauté the cabbage, onion, bell pepper and celery until tender in a skillet that has been coated with no-stick cooking spray. When tender, add the bacon bits, tomato sauce and sugar substitute.

6 servings
Less than 1 fat gram per serving

Snappy Cabbage

1 medium cabbage, coarsely chopped
No-stick cooking spray
3 tablespoons liquid fat-free margarine
3 tablespoons prepared mustard
Light salt and pepper to taste (optional)

Sauté the cabbage in a skillet that has been coated with no-stick cooking spray until it is tender-crisp and slightly browned. Combine the margarine, mustard, light salt and pepper. Add the sauce to the cabbage, cover and cook 5 additional minutes.

6 servings
0 fat grams per serving

Tender-Crisp Cabbage

1 head green cabbage, chopped
No-stick cooking spray
4 tablespoons liquid fat-free margarine
1 packet sugar substitute

Using only the water that clings to it after washing, place the cabbage in a skillet that has been coated with no-stick cooking spray. Sauté over medium heat until the cabbage is tender-crisp and slightly browned. Add the margarine and sugar substitute.

8 servings
0 fat grams per serving

Double Corn Pudding

1 7-ounce package low-fat cornbread mix
1 cup fat-free sour cream
¾ cup fat-free egg substitute
1 15-ounce can whole kernel corn
1 medium onion, finely chopped
1 cup fat-free Cheddar cheese, shredded
Light salt and pepper to taste (optional)
No-stick cooking spray

Combine the cornbread mix, sour cream, egg substitute corn, onion, cheese , light salt and pepper. Place the mixture in a baking dish that has been coated with no-stick cooking spray. Bake for 45 minutes at 350 degrees.

6 servings
3 fat grams per serving

Mexican Corn Casserole

The surprise zip of jalapeno peppers make this casserole different and very good.

1 medium onion, chopped
1 bell pepper, chopped
2 stalks celery, chopped
No-stick cooking spray.
2 cups cooked rice
2 15-ounce cans cream-style corn
1 cup fat-free Cheddar cheese
2 tablespoons fat-free sour cream
1-2 tablespoons chopped jalapeno pepper, depending on
   the degree of hot pepper taste desired
Light salt and pepper to taste (optional)

Sauté the onion, bell pepper and celery in a skillet that has been coated with no-stick cooking spray. When the vegetables are tender, combine them with the remaining ingredients in a casserole dish that has also been coated with no-stick cooking spray. Bake for 30 minutes at 350 degrees.

6 servings
1 fat gram per serving

Skillet Creole Eggplant

If you like eggplant, you will love this spicy dish, Even if you don't like eggplant, give it a try. Eggplant is a vegetable that is versatile, tasty and good for you.

1 large eggplant, unpeeled
1 medium onion, chopped
1 bell pepper, chopped
No-stick cooking spray
1 15-ounce can tomato sauce
1 teaspoon garlic powder
1 teaspoon dried oregano
Light salt and pepper to taste (optional)
Louisiana hot sauce to taste

Sauté the eggplant, onion and pepper in a skillet that has been coated with no-stick cooking spray. When the vegetables are tender, add the tomato sauce, garlic powder, oregano, light salt, pepper and hot sauce. Cover and simmer for 5 minutes.

6 servings
0 fat grams per serving

Chinese-Style Green Bean Casserole

2 15-ounce cans French-style green beans
1 8-ounce can sliced water chestnuts, drained
1 8-ounce can sliced mushrooms, drained
1 15-ounce can bean sprouts, drained
1 8-ounce can bamboo shoots, drained
1 medium onion, finely minced
1 10¾-ounce can 97% fat-free cream of mushroom soup
Light salt and pepper to taste (optional)
No-stick cooking spray

Combine the green beans, water chestnuts, mushrooms, bean sprouts, bamboo shoots, onions, soup, light salt and pepper. Place the mixture in a baking dish that has been coated with no-stick cooking spray. Bake for 30 minutes at 350 degrees.

8 servings
1 fat gram per serving

Quick And Tasty Green Beans

2 15-ounce cans green beans or 2 10-ounce packages frozen
   green beans, cooked and drained
½ cup fat-free sour cream
2 tablespoons dehydrated onion flakes
Light salt and pepper to taste (optional)

Combine all of the ingredients in a saucepan over medium heat. Cook for 5 minutes or until heated through.

8 servings
0 fat grams per serving

Onions! Onions! Onions!

I guess you can tell that I love onions since I use them in lots of recipes. This rich-tasting casserole is about as oniony as you can get!

4 medium onions, coarsely chopped
6 green onions, chopped, including green tops
No-stick cooking spray
1 1-ounce package dehydrated onion soup mix
1 cup skim milk
2 tablespoons all-purpose flour
3 tablespoons liquid fat-free margarine
1 cup fat-free mozzarella cheese, shredded
1 cup low-fat seasoned commercially prepared croutons
Light salt and pepper to taste (optional)

Sauté the onions in a skillet that has been coated with no-stick cooking spray. When they are tender, add the onion soup mix and blend well. Remove from the heat. In a saucepan over medium heat, combine the milk, flour and fat-free liquid margarine. Stir constantly until thickened. Add to the onions and blend well. Add the mozzarella cheese and light salt and pepper to taste. Place the mixture in a baking dish that has been coated with no-stick cooking spray. Sprinkle the croutons on top. Bake for 30 minutes at 350 degrees.

8 servings
Less than 1 fat gram per serving

Mediterranean-Style English Peas

1 medium onion, chopped
No-stick cooking spray
1 cup cracker crumbs, made from fat-free saltines
1 15-ounce can Italian-style chunky tomato sauce
2 15-ounce cans English peas, drained
1 15-ounce can sliced mushrooms, drained
½ cup fat-free Parmesan cheese, grated

Sauté the onions in a skillet that has been coated with no-stick cooking spray until they are tender. Add the cracker crumbs, tomato sauce, English peas, mushrooms and half of the grated Parmesan cheese. Place the mixture in a baking dish that has been coated with no-stick cooking spray. Bake for 30 minutes at 350 degrees. Top with the remaining Parmesan cheese.

8 servings
0 fat grams per serving

Sour Cream Peas

2 15-ounce cans tiny green peas, drained
1 8-ounce can sliced mushrooms, drained
1 cup fat-free sour cream
¼ cup liquid fat-free margarine
Light salt and pepper to taste (optional)

Combine the green peas, mushrooms, sour cream, margarine, light salt and pepper. Place the mixture in a microwave-proof casserole dish and cook on medium for 5 minutes, or place in a saucepan over medium heat on the stovetop and cook until thoroughly warmed.

8 servings
0 fat grams per serving

Hot And Spicy Black-Eyed Peas

1 pound black-eyed peas, soaked overnight and drained
6 cups water
1 medium onion, chopped
1 bell pepper, chopped
2 jalapeno peppers, sliced
1 packet ham or chicken bouillon

In a slow cooker combine the peas, water, onion, peppers and bouillon. Cook on low for 8-10 hours. May also be cooked in a saucepan on the stovetop on medium heat for approximately 1 hour, or until tender.

6 servings
0 fat grams per serving

Barbecued Potatoes

Everyone knows about eating ketchup with French fries, but ketchup and its cousin, barbecue sauce, are terrific with potatoes any way they are cooked.

4 large potatoes, peeled and diced
1 medium onion, chopped
No-stick cooking spray
1 cup fat-free barbecue sauce
1 teaspoon Louisiana-style hot sauce

Sauté the potatoes and onions in a skillet that has been coated with no-stick cooking spray. When they are tender, add the barbecue sauce and hot sauce. Cover and simmer for 5 minutes.

6 servings
0 fat grams per serving

"Butter-Fried" Potatoes

Butter-flavored no-stick cooking spray
5 large baking potatoes, peeled
Butter flavored granules to taste
Liquid fat-free margarine
Louisiana-style hot sauce to taste

Spray a large cookie sheet with low sides with butter-flavored no-stick cooking spray. Cut the potatoes into thin matchsticks or larger-size French fries, depending on preference. Place the potatoes in a single layer on the baking sheet. Very lightly spray the potatoes with butter-flavored no-stick cooking spray. Bake at 425 degrees for 30 minutes, depending upon how brown you like the potatoes. After removing the potatoes from the oven, spray lightly again with the butter-flavored no-stick cooking spray. Sprinkle the potatoes with fat-free, butter-flavored granules to taste. Serve with liquid fat-free margarine combined with a few drops of Louisiana-style hot sauce for dipping.

4 servings
0 fat grams per serving

Fat-Free Mashed Potatoes

This recipe originally appeared in *Live! Don't Diet!* as Mom's Mashed Potatoes. I am repeating it here because several recipes in this book call for prepared fat-free mashed potatoes.

6 medium potatoes, peeled and cut into large chunks
1 ½-ounce package butter-flavored granules
3 tablespoons nonfat dry milk powder
3 tablespoons fat-free sour cream
Light salt and pepper to taste (optional)

Cover the potatoes with water and boil until tender. Drain the potatoes, reserving the cooking liquid. Mash the potatoes, adding the butter-flavored granules, dry milk powder and sour cream. Return as much cooking liquid as needed to achieve desired consistency.

6 servings
0 fat grams per serving

Meal In One Stuffed Potatoes

These make a great side dish but could also serve as an entree with the addition of a little diced low-fat ham or chicken breast.

4 large potatoes, baked
2 tablespoons skim milk
1 10-ounce package frozen chopped broccoli, cooked and
   drained
½ cup fat-free cottage cheese
½ cup fat-free sour cream
1 cup fat-free Cheddar cheese, shredded
4 green onions, chopped, including green tops
4 tablespoons liquid fat-free margarine
Light salt and pepper to taste (optional)
2 tablespoons fat-free Parmesan cheese, grated

Cut the baked potatoes in half horizontally. Scoop the flesh out of each potato half, leaving the skin intact. Mash the potatoes with the milk. Add the broccoli, cottage cheese, sour cream, Cheddar cheese, green onions, liquid margarine and light salt and pepper to taste. The mixture should be firm but not dry. Add additional milk if needed. Stuff the potato skins with the mashed potato mixture. Top with the Parmesan cheese. Bake for 30 minutes at 350 degrees.

8 servings
0 fat grams per serving

Old Country Potato Stuffing

1 medium onion, finely chopped
1 cup celery, finely chopped
No-stick cooking spray
2 cups prepared fat-free mashed potatoes (see recipe index)
1 cup dry bread crumbs
2 tablespoons fat-free liquid margarine
¼ teaspoon sage
¼ cup fat-free egg substitute
Light salt and pepper to taste (optional)

Sauté the onion and celery in a skillet that has been coated with no-stick cooking spray until the vegetables are tender. Combine the sautéed vegetables with the mashed potatoes, bread crumbs, margarine, sage and egg substitute. Add light salt and pepper to taste (optional). Place the mixture in a casserole dish that has been coated with no-stick cooking spray. Bake for 30 minutes at 350 degrees.

4 servings
1 fat gram per serving

My Favorite Sweet Potatoes

4 medium sweet potatoes, peeled, sliced and boiled
½ cup water or skim milk
3 packets sugar substitute
Liquid fat-free margarine

In a mixing bowl, use a potato masher to mash the cooked potatoes until no lumps remain. Add the water or milk and the sugar substitute. Top portions with liquid fat-free margarine to taste.

4 servings
0 fat grams per serving

Sweet Potatoes To Die For

4 large sweet potatoes
Butter-flavored no-stick cooking spray
Fat-free liquid margarine to taste
Cinnamon to taste
Aspartame-based granulated sugar substitute to taste

Lightly coat the potato skins with butter-flavored no-stick cooking spray and place them on a baking pan that has been covered with foil. Bake at 350 degrees for about 2 hours, or until the potatoes are very tender. The actual baking time will depend on the size and shape on the potatoes. Before serving, cut each potato almost in half lengthwise. Squeeze gently to slightly mash the flesh. Add a liberal amount of fat-free liquid margarine to each potato, followed by cinnamon and granulated sugar substitute to taste. Serve immediately.

4 servings
0 fat grams per serving

Easy Baked Rice

1 cup uncooked white rice
1 15-ounce can low-sodium chicken broth
¼ cup water
2 tablespoons Worcestershire sauce
1 package dehydrated onion soup mix
No-stick cooking spray

Combine the rice, chicken broth, water, Worcestershire sauce and onion soup mix in a casserole dish that has been coated with no-stick cooking spray. Cover and bake for 1 ½ hours at 350 degrees.

4 servings
2 fat grams per serving

Autumn Harvest Fruited Rice

1 medium onion, finely chopped
No-stick cooking spray
1 cup uncooked white rice
1 15-ounce can low-sodium, fat-free chicken broth
½ cup plus 2 tablespoons water
½ cup dried apricots, finely chopped
2 tablespoons raisins

In a saucepan that has been coated with no-stick cooking spray, sauté the onion until slightly wilted. Add the rice, chicken broth, water, apricots and raisins. Bring the mixture to a boil, cover and simmer 20 minutes, or until the rice is tender.

4 servings
1 fat gram per serving

Cheesy Spinach Bake

1 cup fat-free egg substitute
1 cup skim milk
1 cup soft breadcrumbs, made from reduced-calorie bread
1 10-ounce package frozen chopped spinach, cooked and
    drained
4 green onions, chopped
¼ cup fat-free Parmesan cheese, grated
1 cup fat-free mozzarella, shredded
Light salt and pepper to taste (optional)
No-stick cooking spray

Combine the egg substitute, milk and breadcrumbs. Let the mixture stand for 5 minutes to moisten the crumbs thoroughly. Add the spinach, onions, Parmesan cheese, mozzarella, light salt and pepper. Place the mixture in a baking dish that has been coated with no-stick cooking spray. Bake for 30 minutes at 350 degrees.

4 servings
Less than 1 fat gram per serving

Deluxe Squash Casserole

1 pound yellow summer squash, boiled, mashed and drained
1 medium onion, finely chopped
10 fat-free saltine crackers, crushed into coarse crumbs
1 cup fat-free Cheddar cheese, shredded
2 tablespoons fat-free sour cream
½ cup fat-free egg substitute
No-stick cooking spray

Combine the squash, onion, cracker crumbs, cheese, sour cream and egg substitute. Place the mixture in a baking dish that has been coated with no-stick cooking spray. Bake for 30 minutes at 350 degrees.

4 servings
0 fat grams per serving

Old-Fashioned Squash Dressing

1 pound yellow summer squash
1 medium onion, finely minced
1 box herb-seasoned stuffing mix prepared according to
   package directions, omitting the margarine
2 tablespoons fat-free sour cream
No-stick cooking spray

Place the squash and onion in a saucepan. Cover with water and simmer until tender. Drain, then mash the squash. Combine all of the ingredients. Place the mixture in a casserole dish that has also been coated with no-stick cooking spray. Bake for 30 minutes at 350 degrees.

6 servings
0 fat grams per serving

Summer Squash Italian-Style

4 yellow summer squash, sliced
4 zucchini, sliced
1 medium onion, sliced
No-stick cooking spray
1 cup fat-free spaghetti sauce
1 tablespoon Parmesan cheese, grated

Sauté the yellow summer squash, zucchini and onion in a skillet that has been coated with no-stick cooking spray. When the vegetables are tender, add the spaghetti sauce. Serve topped with Parmesan cheese.

4 servings
0 fat grams per serving

Skillet-Baked Tomatoes

4 large, firm, ripe tomatoes, halved
No-stick cooking spray
4 tablespoons fat-free Italian salad dressing

Sauté the tomatoes, cut side down in a skillet that has been coated with no-stick cooking spray. When they are slightly brown, turn and spoon 1 tablespoon Italian dressing over the cut side of the tomato halves. Cover and continue cooking for several minutes until warmed through.

8 servings
0 fat grams per serving

Condiments

Barbecue Rub

Many true connoisseurs of barbecue like to coat meat or chicken with a dry marinade before cooking. The traditional tomato-based sauce is added only at the last minute.

¼ cup paprika
¼ cup black pepper, coarsely ground
¼ cup chili powder
2 tablespoons garlic powder
1 tablespoon light salt
2 tablespoons granulated sugar substitute

Combine all ingredients. Store in a tightly covered jar.

1 cup
0 fat grams in the recipe

Bread And Butter Pickles In Minutes

I love bread and butter pickles. They are great with sandwiches or chopped and added to chicken or ham salad. They are also good all by themselves. I like making my own because I can control the amount of salt in them.

¾ cup cider vinegar
1 tablespoon mixed pickling spice
¼ teaspoon light salt
Sugar substitute to equal ⅓ cup sugar
6 cucumbers, preferably unwaxed, sliced
2 medium onions, sliced

Combine the vinegar, the pickling spice and the light salt in a saucepan. Bring to a boil over medium heat. Remove from the heat and add the sugar substitute. Place the vegetables in pint canning jars or in a glass bowl. Pour the vinegar over the vegetables. Store in the refrigerator.

3 pints
0 fat grams in the recipe

Cajun-Style Mayonnaise

Cajun seasoning adds the flair and sparkle that are important in low-fat dishes. This spicy mayonnaise is really good on sandwiches, salads, cold meats or as a dip.

1 cup fat-free mayonnaise
1 tablespoon Cajun seasoning, commercially prepared or
    homemade (see recipe index)
1 tablespoon lemon juice
1 teaspoon garlic powder

Combine the mayonnaise, Cajun seasoning, lemon juice, and garlic powder. Serve chilled.

1 cup
0 fat grams in the recipe

Cajun-Style Seasoning

Popular Cajun-style seasoning is available in most grocery stores. However, it is easily made at home from spices you probably already have on hand.

1 tablespoon light salt
1 tablespoon ground black pepper
2 teaspoons ground red pepper
1 tablespoon dry mustard powder
1 teaspoon garlic powder

Combine the salt, black pepper, red pepper, dry mustard and garlic powder. Store in a tightly capped jar.

4 tablespoons
0 fat grams in the recipe

Country-Style Apple Butter

2 pounds large cooking apples, peeled and chopped
¼ cup cider vinegar
Juice of 1 lemon
1 tablespoon ground cinnamon
1 teaspoon ground cloves
Aspartame-based sugar substitute to equal 2 cups sugar

Combine the apples, vinegar, lemon juice and spices in a saucepan. Cook until the apples are very tender. If there are any whole pieces of apple remaining, puree or mash them until the mixture is smooth. When cool, add the sugar substitute. Store in the refrigerator.

Approximately 2 pints
0 fat grams in the recipe

Dill Sauce For Fish

This recipe is terrific with either fish or shellfish. It is also great as a dressing for potato salad.

¾ cup fat-free mayonnaise
3 tablespoons fat-free sour cream
1 tablespoons skim milk
1 tablespoons dillweed
Light salt to taste

Combine the mayonnaise, sour cream, skim milk, dillweed and light salt. Serve chilled.

1 cup
0 fat grams in the recipe

Extra-Spicy Barbecue Sauce

1 cup ketchup
½ cup cider vinegar
1 tablespoon lemon juice
¼ cup Worcestershire sauce
1 teaspoon garlic powder
1 teaspoon black pepper
1 tablespoon Cajun-style seasoning, commercially prepared or
    homemade (see recipe index)
1 tablespoon liquid smoke
Sugar substitute to equal 2 tablespoons sugar

Combine the ketchup, vinegar, lemon juice, Worcester-shire sauce, spices and liquid smoke in a saucepan. Simmer over medium heat for 15 minutes. Remove from the heat and when cool, add the sugar substitute.

2 cups
0 fat grams in the recipe

Guilt-Free Strawberry Preserves

These preserves are really terrific. While perhaps not as thick as sugary, calorie-laden preserves, they have more intense and wonderful strawberry flavor. A drop or two of red food coloring may be added to deepen the red color. This can double as a great strawberry sauce with angel food cake or fat-free ice cream.

6 cups fresh or frozen strawberries, slightly mashed
1 package pectin made for low-sugar preserves
Aspartame-based sugar substitute to taste

Combine the strawberries and the pectin. Allow to stand 10 minutes. Place in the microwave oven in a deep, microwave-safe bowl. Microwave 5 minutes or until the mixture comes to a boil. Stir, then microwave 4 additional minutes. Stir once again, then microwave 4 more minutes. Allow to cool, then add sugar substitute to taste. Pour into canning jars or plastic freezer containers. Store in the refrigerator or freezer.

3 pints
0 fat grams in the recipe

Homemade Crispy Coating For Chicken

This is a homemade version of the coating mixes sold for oven-frying chicken. It is also good as a coating for oven-fried vegetables. Just spray the chicken or vegetables with no-stick cooking spray and dip in the coating mix. Spray the coated pieces again lightly with the no-stick cooking spray and bake at 425 degrees.

2 cups fine, dry breadcrumbs
½ cup all-purpose flour
2 teaspoons light salt
1 tablespoon poultry seasoning
1 teaspoon black pepper
2 teaspoons garlic powder

Combine the breadcrumbs, flour, light salt, poultry seasoning, black pepper and garlic powder. Store in a tightly covered jar.

2 ¾ cups
0 fat grams in the recipe

Honey Mustard Sauce

This makes a really good dip, salad dressing, sandwich spread or sauce for grilled chicken. This recipe is a really terrific one—it has only three inexpensive ingredients, can be made in seconds and can be used a number of ways. You can't ask for more than that!

½ cup Dijon-style mustard
½ cup fat-free mayonnaise
2 tablespoons honey

Combine the Dijon mustard, mayonnaise and honey. Can be served chilled or warm.

4 servings
0 fat grams per serving

Peach Pie Preserves

I had a basket of fresh peaches on hand last summer that had gotten very ripe. I am a terribly lazy cook. Rather than get my act together and peel those peaches, I decided to experiment by leaving the peels on. If my experiment hadn't worked, I guess I would have had to change the name of the recipe to Fuzzy Peach Preserves. However, they really turned out great. There was no sign of peach fuzz and the peels on the peaches were not even noticeable.

12-15 very ripe peaches, chopped
1 box pectin made for low-sugar preserves
Aspartame-based sugar substitute to taste
Nutmeg to taste
Cinnamon to taste

Slightly mash the peaches. Combine them with the pectin and allow to stand for 10 minutes. Bring to a boil over medium heat. Lower the heat and allow to simmer 10 minutes. Remove from the heat. When the preserves have cooled slightly, add the sugar substitute and spices to taste. Pour into canning jars or plastic freezer containers. Store in the refrigerator or freezer.

3 pints
0 fat grams in the recipe

Piquant Beet Relish

I happen to like beets but even those who don't may like this relish. It is good with dried beans.

3 15-ounce cans sliced beets, chopped
1 medium onion, chopped
½ medium green cabbage, chopped
½ teaspoon light salt (optional)
1 ½ cups cider vinegar
Sugar substitute to equal ¾ cup sugar

Combine the beets, onion, cabbage, salt and vinegar in a medium saucepan. Bring to a boil, then simmer 10 minutes. Remove from the heat and when cool, add the sugar substitute. Store in canning jars or a covered glass dish in the refrigerator.

3 pints
0 fat grams in the recipe

Zippy Mayonnaise

Even if you don't care for fat-free mayonnaise, you will like this spicy version. It is good as a sandwich spread or as a dressing for green salads, pasta salads, or potato salad.

1 cup fat-free mayonnaise
3 tablespoons prepared mustard
2 teaspoons lemon juice
1 teaspoon Louisiana-style hot sauce

Combine the mayonnaise, mustard, lemon juice and hot sauce. Serve chilled.

1 ¼ cups
0 fat grams in the recipe

Desserts

Angel's Wing Cake

This cake is so light and delicious I could eat it all by myself. It makes a nice fat-free birthday cake since it is very pretty.

1 8-ounce container fat-free whipped topping, thawed
1 small (4 serving-size) box vanilla fat-free, sugar-free pudding mix
1 8-ounce can juice-packed crushed pineapple, drained
1 commercially prepared angel food cake

In a mixing bowl, combine the whipped topping, the dry pudding mix and the fruit. Fold the ingredients together gently. Slice the cake horizontally into 3 equal layers. Frost the top and sides of one layer with the whipped topping mixture. Add the second layer, then the third, frosting the top and sides of each.

12 servings
0 fat grams per serving

Autumn Fruit Bake

This is a wonderful dessert for cool weather, I guess because the dried fruit seems like fall or winter. It is good topped with fat-free whipped topping or ice cream. Leave off the cookie topping and it could be served as a fruit compote with ham or turkey.

1 15-ounce can juice-packed pear halves, drained and chopped
   (reserve juice)
1 15-ounce can juice-packed peaches, drained and chopped
   (reserve juice)
1 cup mixed dried fruit (prunes, apples and apricots)
1 15-ounce can light cherry pie filling
4 fat-free or low-fat oatmeal cookies, crumbled
No-stick cooking spray

Combine the reserved juice with the dried fruit. Cover and microwave for 5 minutes. Drain and discard any remaining liquid. Combine the pears, peaches, dried fruit and cherry pie filling. Top with the crumbled cookies. Spray the cookies lightly with no-stick cooking spray. Bake for 30 minutes at 350 degrees.

8 servings
0 fat grams per serving, if fat-free cookies are used

Banana Pudding In A Cone

Thank goodness for ice cream cones. They make ice cream a portable treat. Now they do the same thing for another favorite dessert—banana pudding. An old-fashioned ice cream cone has only a trace of fat and only 20 calories. They can be used in a variety of creative ways that appeal to kids, as well as the kid in all of us. Sundaes in cones (fat-free frozen yogurt, low-fat sundae topping and fat-free whipped topping), pudding in cones or even cupcakes in cones (light cake mix baked in flat-bottomed cones) are just some of the possibilities.

1 small (4 serving-size) box fat-free, sugar-free banana-
    flavored pudding mix
2 cups skim milk
1 medium banana, thinly sliced
4 old-fashioned, flat-bottomed ice cream cones
4 tablespoons fat-free whipped topping

Combine the pudding mix and milk. Blend well. When it has thickened, layer pudding and banana slices in each cone. Top with a tablespoon of fat-free whipped topping.

4 servings
Less than 1 fat gram per serving

Banana Shortcake

Light cake mixes are now available in many flavors. They have substantially less fat than conventional cake mixes and taste just as good. You will never notice that this tasty shortcake is missing anything, especially since it tastes so rich and creamy. It couldn't be any better.

1 light white or yellow cake mix
½ cup fat-free egg substitute
1 large (8 serving-size) box fat-free, sugar-free vanilla pudding
    mix
4½ cups skim milk
2 medium-size ripe bananas

Prepare the cake mix according to package directions, using fat-free egg substitute instead of eggs. Bake in a 9" x 13" baking dish that has been coated with no-stick cooking spray. Baking time will depend on package directions. Meanwhile, combine the pudding and the skim milk. The pudding should be the consistency of a custard sauce. Add additional milk if needed to achieve desired consistency. Shortly before serving, thinly slice the bananas. Cut the cake into twelve equal squares. For each serving, place one cake square on an individual serving plate. Top with a portion of the sauce and banana slices.

12 servings
Less than 2 fat grams per serving

Cherry Cobbler Cake

This is a tasty combination—the fruity filling of cobbler topped by the moist tenderness of cake. For all its simplicity, this is a big hit when I take it to potluck dinners.

2 15-ounce cans light cherry pie filling
No-stick cooking spray
1 light yellow or white cake mix
½ cup fat-free egg substitute

Pour the cherry pie filling into a 9" x 13" baking dish that has been coated with no-stick cooking spray. Prepare the cake mix according to package directions, using egg substitute instead of eggs. Pour the prepared cake batter over the fruit filling. Bake for 30 minutes at 350 degrees.

12 servings
2 fat grams per serving

Cherry Cream Cheese Pie

Commercially prepared pie crusts can be fairly low in fat if you read labels carefully and choose the right brand. Pastry crusts average 8 fat grams per serving if you divide your pie into eight servings. Graham cracker crusts average 6 grams for the same size serving. Lower-fat prepared graham cracker crusts are now in grocery stores. They have only 3 fat grams per serving.

1 small (4 serving-size) box fat-free, sugar-free vanilla
    pudding mix
1 ½ cups skim milk
1 8-ounce package fat-free cream cheese, softened
¼ teaspoon vanilla extract
6 packets aspartame-based sugar substitute
1 lower-fat graham cracker pie crust
1 15-ounce can light cherry pie filling

In a mixing bowl, combine the pudding mix and skim milk. Blend until the pudding mix is dissolved. Set aside. In a separate mixing bowl, combine the cream cheese, vanilla extract and sugar substitute. Gently fold the pudding and cream cheese together. When thoroughly combined, pour the mixture into the graham cracker pie crust. Spread the cherry pie filling over the cream cheese layer. Chill for several hours.

8 servings
3 fat grams per serving

Chocolate Decadence

Never leave me alone with this dessert. There won't be any left if I get my hands on it.

1 large (8 serving-size) box fat-free, sugar-free chocolate fudge
    pudding mix
4 cup cold skim milk
1 light cake mix, chocolate or chocolate fudge flavor
½ cup fat-free egg substitute
No-stick cooking spray
6 fat-free or low-fat chocolate cream-filled cookies
1 cup fat-free whipped topping

Combine the pudding mix and skim milk. Stir well. Refrigerate until needed. Meanwhile prepare the cake mix according to package directions, using the egg substitute instead of eggs. Bake the cake in a 9" x 13" pan that has been coated with no-stick cooking spray. The baking time will depend on package directions. When the cake has cooled, cut into 1" wide slices. Chop the cookies into coarse crumbs. In a large serving dish, preferably clear glass, place a layer of cake slices, followed by a layer of pudding. Sprinkle the pudding with chopped cookie crumbs. Repeat the layers until all of the cake and pudding has been used. Reserve some cookie crumbs for the top of the dessert. After all of the cake and pudding has been used, spread the whipped topping over the top. Sprinkle with the reserved cookie crumbs.

12 servings
2 fat grams per serving

Cranberry Upside Down Cake

The surprise ingredient in this delicious recipe is the cranberry sauce. It develops a mellow richness in the cooking process. Few people would even guess that it's just good old cranberry sauce in disguise.

2 15-ounce cans whole berry cranberry sauce
1 15-ounce can juice-packed crushed pineapple, undrained
1 light yellow or white cake mix
½ cup fat-free egg substitute
No-stick cooking spray

Combine the cranberry sauce and the crushed pineapple. Spread the mixture into a 9" x 13" baking dish that has been coated with no-stick cooking spray. Prepare the cake mix according to package directions, using the egg substitute instead of the eggs called for in the recipe. Pour the cake mix over the cranberry layer. Bake for 30 minutes at 350 degrees.

12 servings
Less than 2 fat grams per serving

Desperation Pie In An Instant

Here's another taste-alike. This is what I often make when I have a craving for apple pie and there is no low-fat apple pie around. It's a pretty effective way to satisfy that sweet tooth in a quick and healthy manner. You get crunch from the rice cake and the delicious taste of apples and cinnamon—the same taste sensations that make real apple pie so wonderful.

For each "pie":
1 caramel rice cake
2 tablespoons unsweetened applesauce
Cinnamon to taste
Granulated aspartame-based sugar substitute

Spread the applesauce on the rice cake. Sprinkle with the cinnamon and sugar substitute to taste. Can be topped with fat-free vanilla frozen yogurt if desired. Serve immediately.

1 serving
0 fat grams per serving

Fabulous Tropical Frozen Yogurt

Isn't it great that ice cream and frozen yogurt are now available in a fat-free, sugar-free form? It is fun to experiment by using your own favorite extras to create a personalized frozen treat. The possibilities are limitless.

½ gallon fat-free, sugar-free, vanilla-flavored frozen yogurt, softened
2 teaspoons coconut extract (or more, according to taste)
1 15-ounce can juice-packed crushed pineapple, drained
1 8-ounce can juice-packed mandarin oranges, drained

In a mixing bowl, combine the softened frozen yogurt, coconut extract, pineapple and mandarin oranges. Place the mixture in a freezer-proof storage container with a sealable lid and re-freeze. Let stand at room temperature for 5 minutes before serving.

16 servings
0 fat grams per serving

Fat-Free, Sugar-Free Fudge Truffles

Truffles are a favorite of candy lovers. Unfortunately, they are loaded with sugar and fat. Never fear! Here are two recipes for truffles that can satisfy your your sweet tooth and your healthy lifesyle. To be fancy, place in ruffled paper candy cups.

3-4 tablespoons cocoa powder
10-12 packets aspartame-based sugar substitute
8 ounces fat-free cream cheese, softened

Gradually add the cocoa powder and sugar substitute to the softened cream cheese. Taste after adding three tablespoons of cocoa. At this point the candies will have the taste of bittersweet chocolate. Add additional cocoa powder and/or sugar substitute if you wish. Chill until firm. Shape the mixture into small balls, then roll in additional cocoa powder mixed with an equal amount of sugar substitute. Store in the refrigerator.

24 candies, 0 fat grams per candy

Cheesecake Truffles

8 ounces fat-free cream cheese softened
½ teaspoon vanilla, coconut, orange or almond extract
12 packets aspartame-based sugar substitute
¼ cup graham cracker crumbs
Dash cinnamon

Combine the softened cream cheese with the extract and 10 packets of sugar substitute. Taste and add more sugar substitute or extract if desired. Chill the mixture until firm. Meanwhile, combine the graham cracker crumbs, 2 packets of sugar substitute and a dash of cinnamon. Shape the cream cheese mixture into small balls and roll each ball in the graham cracker crumbs. Store in the refrigerator.

24 candies, 0 fat grams per candy

Guilt-Free No-Bake Cheesecake

One of the world's most beloved desserts is unfortunately one of the most fat-laden. There are many recipes for low-fat cheesecake around but they often still contain heaps of sugar. Here is the recipe that has no fat, no sugar and as an added bonus, does not have to be baked.

3 tablespoons cornflake crumbs combined with 1 packet sugar
    substitute and ¼ teaspoon cinnamon
4 8-ounce packages fat-free cream cheese, softened
Aspartame-based sugar substitute to equal 1 cup sugar
1 packet unflavored gelatin
1 ¼ cups water, divided
1 teaspoon each vanilla, butter, coconut and orange extract

Coat an 8 inch or 9 inch springform pan with no-stick cooking spray. Sprinkle with the cornflake crumb mixture and shake the pan to coat the bottom and sides evenly. Reserve a bit of the mixture to top the cheesecake if desired. Add the sugar substitute to the softened creamed cheese. In a measuring cup, combine the unflavored gelatin with ¼ cup cold water. Allow it to stand for 2 minutes, then microwave for 1 minute. Make sure the gelatin is completely dissolved. Add the gelatin to the cream cheese mixture, followed by the remaining 1 cup of water and the extract. Blend well, preferably with a hand mixer or whisk. Chill until firm.

6 servings
0 fat grams per serving

Heavenly Ambrosia

2 15-ounce cans juice-packed pineapple tidbits, drained
4 medium oranges, peeled, seeded and sectioned
2 medium bananas, thinly sliced
1 cup miniature marshmallows
1 cup fat-free vanilla-flavored yogurt
1 small (4-serving-size) box fat-free, sugar-free vanilla
  pudding mix
1 cup skim milk

In a serving bowl, combine the pineapple, oranges, bananas and marshmallows. In a separate bowl, combine the yogurt, pudding mix and milk. Blend well. Combine the yogurt mixture with the fruit mixture and serve immediately. Serve alone in stemmed glasses or over fat-free pound cake or angel food cake.

8 servings
0 fat grams per serving

Kind Of Pie

When I want pie, I often make a taste-alike version that will make me happy without having a whole pie around to tempt me. My very favorite pie is lemon icebox. I like the smooth creamy tartness of the filling and the crunchy texture of the graham cracker crust. While this recipe is for a lemon icebox taste-alike, this parfait can satisfy your desire for almost kind of pie. Just substitute your own favorite filling. The real appeal of pie is the sweetness of a fruit or cream filling combined with crunch. You get that here, along with a simplicity of preparation that can't be beat.

1 small (4 serving-size) box fat-free, sugar-free vanilla pudding mix
1 ¾ cups skim milk
2 tablespoons lemon juice
Sugar substitute to taste
½ cup graham cracker crumbs
4 tablespoons fat-free whipped topping

Combine the pudding mix and milk. Add the lemon juice and sugar substitute to taste. For each serving, layer the pudding mixture and graham cracker crumbs in individual parfaits or serving dishes. Top with the whipped topping.

4 servings
0 fat grams per serving

Light And Fruity Orange Sherbet

This is also great made with other fruit juices. Try pineappple juice, grape juice or combined juices, like orange-pineapple.

2 cups unsweetened orange juice
⅓ cup non-fat dry milk powder
3 packets aspartame-based artificial sweetener

Combine the orange juice, milk powder and sweetener. Blend thoroughly. Pour the mixture into a baking pan and freeze until slightly firm. Remove from the freezer and beat until smooth and creamy. Return to the freezer. Allow to stand a few minutes at room temperature before serving.

4 servings
0 fat grams per serving

Old-Fashioned Peach Dumplings

Dumplings lend themselves to all kinds of delicious adaptations, including dessert. They are also a terrific comfort food. Fat-free, sugar-free vanilla frozen yogurt is great served on top of individual servings.

2 15-ounce cans sliced juice-packed peaches, juice reserved
4 cups water
1 13.5-ounce package fat-free flour tortillas, cut into 1" squares
8 packets aspartame-based sugar substitute
1 tablespoon cinnamon

Combine the reserved peach juice and water in a saucepan. Bring to a boil over medium heat. Gradually add the tortilla squares, stirring frequently, so that they won't stick together. Cook for 10 minutes or until the dumplings lose their doughy consistency. Add the peaches, 6 packets sugar substitute and a dash of cinnamon. In a separate bowl, combine the remaining sugar substitute and cinnamon. Place the dumplings in individual serving bowls and top with a bit of the cinnamon mixture. Serve immediately,

8 servings
0 fat grams per serving

Pancake Cake

While not exactly a company dessert, this a distant cousin of the elaborate gourmet treat Crepes Suzette. Low-fat packaged pancake mix or frozen pancakes can be used if you prefer.

2 ¼ cups all-purpose flour
4 teaspoons baking powder
1 teaspoon light salt
2 cups skim milk
¼ cup fat-free egg substitute
4 tablespoons fat-free cottage cheese
Butter-flavored no-stick cooking spray
1 cup low-sugar orange marmalade

Orange Sauce:
1 cup orange juice
1 tablespoon cornstarch
3 packets aspartame-based sugar substitute

Combine the flour, baking powder, salt, skim milk and egg substitute. On a griddle that has been coated with no-stick cooking spray, pour enough batter to form an 8" pancake. When bubbles form on the uncooked side, turn and cook for 2 additional minutes. Repeat until all of the pancake batter has been used. Spread each layer with a generous coating of orange marmalade, then stack them to resemble a cake. To make the sauce, combine the orange juice and cornstarch. Bring to a boil over medium heat until the mixture thickens. Add the sugar substitute. Top with the warm orange sauce.

4 servings
0 fat grams per serving

Punchbowl Cake

This is another flexible dessert recipe that is popular around our house. You can use low-fat yellow or white cake or angel food cake and just about any fruit that suits your fancy. I like to use purchased angel food cake for several reasons. It is fat-free, delicious, and best of all, I don't have to bake it! This is very pretty when served in a glass punchbowl or serving dish.

1 large (8 serving-size) box fat-free, sugar-free vanilla pudding mix
4 cups skim milk
1 large commercially prepared angel food cake ring, torn into bite-size pieces
1 15-ounce can juice-packed sliced peaches, drained and chopped
1 8-ounce can juice-packed crushed pineapple, drained
3 large ripe bananas, thinly sliced
1 15-ounce can light cherry pie filling
1 cup fat-free whipped topping

Combine the pudding mix and milk. Set aside to thicken. In a large glass serving bowl, place ¼ of the cake pieces, followed by the peaches, then ¼ of the pudding. Repeat the layers, using the pineapple. Repeat again, using the sliced bananas. Top the bananas with the last layer of cake, followed by pudding, then the cherry pie filling. Garnish with dollops of whipped topping.

12 servings
Less than 1 fat-gram per serving

Rich And Creamy Cheesecake

Here is another tasty no-bake cheesecake without fat or sugar. Use any type crushed fat-free cereal to make the crust and any flavor fat-free pudding mix.

6 tablespoons fat-free nutty nugget-type cereal
Dash cinnamon
15 packets aspartame-based sugar substitute, divided
No-stick cooking spray
¼ cup boiling water
1 packet unflavored gelatin
1 small (4 serving-size) box fat-free, sugar-free vanilla
    pudding mix
1½ cups skim milk
3 8-ounce packages fat-free cream cheese, softened
1 teaspoon vanilla extract

Combine the cereal, cinnamon and 3 packets sugar substitute. Coat an 8" or 9" springform pan or pie plate with no-stick cooking spray. Pour the cereal mixture into the pan and shake the pan gently to coat the bottom and sides with the cereal mixture. In a measuring cup, combine the boiling water and gelatin. Stir well to dissolve the gelatin. Allow to cool to room temperature. In a mixing bowl, combine the pudding mix and milk. Add the cooled gelatin mixture and blend well. Gently fold the pudding mixture into the softened cream cheese. Add 12 packets sugar substitute and the vanilla extract. Pour the cream cheese mixture over the crust. Cover and chill for at least 4 hours.

8 servings
0 fat grams per serving

Taste-Alike Instant Dutch Apple Cobbler

I am a sucker for Dutch apple pie. Lots of us are. While it is usually made with hefty amounts of butter and sugar, we don't have to do without it just because we are eating healthy. We can make a taste-alike. Let's analyze the taste we love in Dutch apple pie. There is the taste of apples, cinnamon and sugar combined with the sweet crunch of streusel. All we have to do is use sugar substitute for the sugar, while low-fat granola cereal makes a dandy substitute for the streusel.

2 15-ounce cans sliced, unsweetened apples
Sugar substitute to taste
1 teaspoon apple pie spice
4 tablespoons low-fat granola cereal

Combine the apples, the sugar substitute and apple pie spice in a microwave-safe baking dish. Cover loosely with plastic wrap and microwave on high power for 5 minutes. Remove and evenly sprinkle the granola over the fruit. Return to the microwave for 30 seconds on high power. Serve plain or topped with fat-free, sugar-free frozen yogurt.

Variation: Use canned, sliced peaches or low-sugar commercially prepared fruit pie filling.

4 servings
1 fat gram per serving

Caloric/Fat Analysis Of The Recipes

I don't count calories because it reminds me too much of dieting. That is why I list only the fat grams per serving on the page with my recipes. However, monitoring the calories is important to some people. The nutritional information below is based on individual servings and is rounded off to the nearest whole number.

Breakfast:	kcal	total fat
Potato Crusted Breakfast Pie	144	2
Ham and Cheese Casserole	220	5
Cottage Cheese Pancakes	199	0
Cheesy Breakfast Burrito	177	0
Appetizers:		
Baked Bean Dip	108	1
Chunky Bean Spread	123	0
Don't Give Up The Chip	114	0
Heavenly Fruit/Nut Spread	128	0
Herbed Cream Cheese Spread	32	0
Snappy Crackers	23	0
Tangy Shrimp Spread	105	1
Soups:		
Almost Effortless Ravioli Stew	241	0
Chunky Potato Soup	117	0
Hearty White Chili	371	2
Smoky Split Pea Soup	241	1
Terrific Taco Soup	392	4
Vegetable Soup With A Kick	202	2
Warm/Cozy Cream Of Tomato	183	0
Salads:		
Baked Bean Salad	298	1
Cheesy Italian Potato Salad	91	0
Cool Summer Salad	198	3
Crisp Apple Slaw	93	0
Crunchy Apple Salad	166	0
Delicious Layered Slaw	81	0
Delightful Frozen Fruit Salad	60	0
Holiday Cranberry Salad	50	0
Jellied Fresh Fruit Salad	56	0
Killer Salsa Salad	29	0
Kind Of Greek Salad	50	0
Mexican Spinach Salad	80	0
Secret Tuna Salad	88	1
Snappy Green Bean Salad	59	0
Summer In A Bowl	132	0
Beef:		
Acapulco Rice	339	3
Baked Beef/Pasta Supreme	400	4
Barbecue Pie	285	5
Chili Mountain	468	4

Beef-Continued:	*kcal*	*total fat*
Country Style Butterbean Pie	319	3
Creamy Pasta Casserole	267	3
Dinnertime Sloppy Joes	149	2
Extra Easy Eye Of Round Roast	183	6
Gourmet Steak	251	6
Onion Baked Steak	250	5
Pizza-Macaroni Style	323	3
Ken's Quick Stuffed Peppers	332	4
Slow Cooker Oriental Beef	295	4
Spaghetti With A Difference	384	4
Steak In A Stew	372	5
Steak Teriyaki	189	5
Tasty Tamale Pie	124	2
Chicken:		
Barbecued Chicken Casserole	248	4
Basic Lemon-Herb Chicken	134	6
Chicken Italian	173	6
Chunky Chicken Hash	278	5
Creamy Chicken Casserole	300	5
Crispy Oven Chicken	181	5
Ham And Cheese Chicken	139	4
Chicken Picante	132	4
Mexican Grilled Chicken	100	4
Pasta Jambalaya	251	5
Peachy Chicken Delight	149	4
Piquant Barbecued Chicken	124	6
Quick And Tender Turkey	170	3
Rich And Creamy Chicken	175	3
Slow Cooker Chicken	154	5
Cranberry Chicken	260	4
Spectacular Stuffed Chicken	299	5
Turkey Divan Casserole	241	4
Uptown Chicken Hollandaise	202	4
Pork:		
American Dinner Pie	197	0
Ashley's Chinese Burritos	379	1
Autumn Pork Tenderloin	355	4
Baked Pork Supreme	219	3
Busy Day Ham/Dumplings	384	2
Country-Style Pork	184	3
Creole Smoked Sausage	163	3
Deluxe Ham/Cheese Casserole	257	2
Deluxe Stuffed Wieners	352	0
Extra Lazy Sweet/Sour Ham	400	2
Glorified Ham/Rice Casserole	320	2
Ham Casserole Deluxe	284	2
Potato Stuffed Wieners	107	0
Red Beans And Rice Casserole	284	1

Pork:	*kcal*	*total fat*
Simple, Crispy Pork Cutlets	128	3
Slow Cooker Dinner	278	2
Sautéed Smoked Sausage	70	1
Smoked Sausage Dinner	188	2
Stick To Your Ribs Ham	204	2
Stroganoff With Ham	336	3
Tempting Tenderloin	325	4
Seafood:		
Baked Fish In A Hurry	200	3
Chinese-Style Sesame Shrimp	205	5
Crispy Sesame Broiled Scallops	193	8
Crunchy Tuna	254	1
Mandarin Baked Snapper Fillets	240	3
Oven Baked Shrimp Jambalaya	287	2
Oven Fried Fish	244	2
Quick And Spicy Fish Fillets	189	2
Saucy Shrimp And Pasta	289	2
Scallop Sauté	113	2
Shrimp Stroganoff	358	3
Sunday Salmon Loaf	187	4
Tempting Baked Fish	328	3
Tuna/Rice Casserole	235	1
Zesty Fish Scampi	165	2
Meatless Entrees:		
Baked Egg Foo Young	51	1
Lasagna In Cream Sauce	249	1
Creamy Fettucini	220	1
Easy Cheesy Pie	210	0
Old-Fashioned Dumplings	305	1
Rich Ravioli Casserole	416	0
Shortcut Baked Lasagna	251	1
South Of The Border Tacos	364	2
Terrific Potato Enchiladas	248	0
Breads:		
Baked Apple Fritters	71	0
Baked Banana Fritters	80	0
Blueberry Bran Muffins	96	0
Classic Corn Fritters	32	0
Classic Muffins	95	0
Comforting Cornbread	191	1
Kind Of Donuts	33	0
Lazy Day Apple Muffins	120	1
Mom's Yeast Cornbread	226	1
Onion Flatbread	125	0
Poor Folk's Pizza	136	1
Quick Apple Muffins	46	0
Vegetables:		
Coffee Baked Beans	127	0

Vegetables-Continued:	kcal	total fat
Mom's Broccoli Casserole	15	1
Sautéed Broccoli Oriental	22	0
Brussels Sprouts	65	0
Skillet Cabbage Supreme	68	1
Snappy Cabbage	37	0
Tender Crisp Cabbage	35	0
Double Corn Pudding	261	3
Mexican Corn Casserole	238	1
Skillet Eggplant	75	0
Chinese Green Beans	44	1
Quick And Tasty Green Beans	41	0
Onions Onions Onions	109	1
Mediterranean English Peas	109	0
Sour Cream Peas	91	0
Hot And Spicy Black Eyed Peas	170	0
Barbecued Potatoes	95	0
"Butter-Fried" Potatoes	105	0
Fat-Free Mashed Potatoes	111	0
Meal In One Stuffed Potatoes	150	0
Old Country Potato Stuffing	144	1
My Favorite Sweet Potatoes	151	0
Sweet Potatoes To Die For	175	0
Easy Baked Rice	234	2
Autumn Harvest Fruited Rice	270	1
Cheesy Spinach Bake	200	1
Deluxe Squash Casserole	74	0
Old-Fashioned Squash	318	0
Summer Squash Italian	59	0
Skillet-Baked Tomatoes	29	0
Condiments:		
Barbecue Rub	5	0
Bread And Butter Pickles	19	0
Cajun-Style Mayonnaise	13	0
Cajun-Style Seasoning	6	0
Country-Style Apple Butter	17	0
Dill Sauce For Fish	35	0
Extra-Spicy Barbecue Sauce	19	0
Guilt-Free Strawberry Preserves	11	0
Homemade Crispy Coating	74	0
Honey Mustard Sauce	75	0
Peach Pie Preserves	13	0
Piquant Beet Relish	84	0
Zippy Mayonnaise	10	0
Desserts:		
Angel's Wing Cake	189	0
Autumn Fruit Bake	75	0
Banana Pudding In A Cone	113	1
Banana Shortcake	173	2

Desserts-Continued:	*kcal*	*total fat*
Cherry Cobbler Cake	186	2
Cherry Cream Cheese Pie	203	3
Chocolate Decadence	182	2
Cranberry Upside Down Cake	201	2
Desperation Pie In An Instant	59	0
Fabulous Frozen Yogurt	205	0
Fat-Free Fudge Truffles	12	0
Cheesecake Truffles	18	0
Guilt-Free Cheesecake	163	0
Heavenly Ambrosia	174	0
Kind Of Pie	124	0
Light And Fruity Sherbet	86	0
Old Fashioned Dumplings	203	0
Pancake Cake	185	0
Punchbowl Cake	231	1
Rich And Creamy Cheesecake	48	0
Taste Alike Apple Cobbler	153	1

Recipe Index